# Praise for *Master Your Stress, Re*

"Our body has a tremendous ability to heal—if we just give it a chance. Unfortunately, the relentless environmental, emotional and life stress sabotages this ability. Thank you Dr. Doni for such an authoritative, but easily read and applied resource for everyone."

—**Dr. Joe Pizzorno, ND**, co-author of *Encyclopedia of Natural Medicine* and founding president of Bastyr University

"Stress is not one size fits all. It is different for every individual. And if you don't approach it correctly, you can make it worse! Dr. Doni has identified unique Stress Types and the right support for each, so you can find your personalized stress cure and turn your stress into your advantage!"

—**JJ Virgin, CNS**, *New York Times* bestselling author of *The Virgin Diet*

"Dr. Doni Wilson has focused on the importance of stress reduction for years. She has recognized the central role it plays in nearly every symptom and disease and found innovative ways to help people master their stress. This book represents the culmination of years of her research and clinical experience. I'm confident that the advice in it will help anyone who has recognized that stress is their core issue."

—**Alan Christianson, NMD, FABNE**, *New York Times* bestselling author of the *Thyroid Reset Diet*

"Stress affects each of us, but not in the same way. To recover from stress and burnout, we have to first understand how stress impacts us. Then we can reverse the health issues caused by stress and improve our longevity. Thanks to Dr. Doni Wilson for putting this information together so we can all benefit."

—**Dr. Trevor Cates**, author of the *USA Today* bestseller *Clean Skin From Within*

"Dr. Doni Wilson has timed this book perfectly—such stressful times with new big stressors in our world at large in addition to the more common stressors that we face daily. This book will clarify the mechanisms that occur in the body to create a cascade of consequences related to stress including fatigue, anxiety, and insomnia, and then she teaches us and gives instructions on how we can recover some ground and feel better again. She offers specific, insightful, as well as practical and sound strategies for solutions with lifestyle management, botanicals, and nutraceuticals."

—**Tori Hudson, ND,** author of *Women's Encyclopedia of Natural Medicine*

"Outstanding! *Master Your Stress, Reset Your Health* is a game-changer in assessing and treating stress-related illness. The cutting-edge, personalized information in this book can help you recover your health with proven natural therapies."

—**Dr. Mark Stengler,** bestselling author of *Prescription for Natural Cures*

"Dr. Doni Wilson is an expert in her field and one of the most dependable voices that I actively seek out, for both my family's health and the health of my clients."
—**Dr. Debi Silber,** founder of
The Post Betrayal Transformation Institute (PBT)

"Stress is one of the great agers of our body, inside and out. While it's easy to tell someone they should reduce their stress level, how can it practically be done? Nationally-recognized naturopathic physician Dr. Doni Wilson has written a wonderful book that gives practical, actionable advice that anyone can follow to reduce their stress and live longer, healthier, and happier lives."
—**Anthony Youn, MD, FACS,** America's Holistic
Plastic Surgeon® and author of *The Age Fix*

"We all need this book! *Master Your Stress, Reset Your Health* by my colleague Dr. Wilson is an excellent step-by-step guide to undoing what stress does to us. I have been in medicine since the 1970's and can unequivocally state that stress and its effects on us creates more basis for chronic health issues than any other trigger. Please use this book and share it with your friends and loved ones to start on the path to healing."
—**Dr. Paul S. Anderson,** Physician and author of
*The Natural Physician's Healing Therapies*

"As an insightful clinician, I actively seek out to provide a blueprint for how to get our stress levels better managed and provide the solutions to get my patients' health back on track . . . *Master Your Stress, Reset Your Health* is a must read!"
—**Cynthia Thurlow,** Nurse practitioner, TEDx speaker, and author of
*Intermittent Fasting Transformation: IF45* (publishes March 2022)

"After a lifetime of pushing my body on the playing field and the stage, I've discovered how important it is to manage my stress, and to value recovery. Dr. Doni Wilson gives the exact blueprint for champions who want to give their bodies the proper stress support, and how to de-stress in a systematic and strategic way that builds resilience."
—**Bo Eason,** NFL All-Pro, in-demand speaker,
and 7-time bestselling author

"Dr. Doni is truly an expert on diagnosing and treating the many impacts on health that stress causes. I recommend *Master Your Stress, Reset Your Health* to many of my patients. She has written about her personal and professional experience in easy to understand language, with helpful examples and metaphors."
—**Michael Traub, ND, FABNO**, clinician, researcher, and author

"Stress can chip away at your quality of life and lead to a host of health issues like high blood pressure, low libido, and anxiety. In *Master Your Stress, Reset Your Health* you'll be able to identify your stress type and get the solutions you need to amplify your health and happiness."

**—Dr. Jolene Brighten, NMD, FABNE,**
and bestselling author of *Beyond the Pill*

"Dr. Doni Wilson changed my life—and my son Isaiah's life—15 years ago when she helped us using the protocol she describes in *Master Your Stress, Reset Your Health*. I'm so happy for everyone to now have access to her effective, transformative approach."

**—Silvana Nardone,** author of the bestselling *Cooking for Isaiah: Gluten-Free & Dairy-Free Recipes for Easy, Delicious Meals*

"*Master Your Stress, Reset Your Health* is a *must-read* if stress and the effects of stress (e.g., high blood pressure, digestive issues, muscle tension) are taking you down. Information is clearly presented and the strategies for addressing stress are well thought out, practical, effective, and easy to implement. Using them, you're bound to experience less stress and a greater sense of well-being. Thank you, Dr. Doni Wilson, for gifting us with so many resources and your C.A.R.E. approach!"

**—Dr. Joan Rosenberg**, Psychologist and Author of
*90 Seconds to a Life You Love*

"*Master Your Stress, Reset Your Health* is a wealth of knowledge and I am grateful that the public has access to it. Dr. Wilson's writing will provide comfort and advice to all those who need it. In the book Dr. Wilson outlines the five most common Stress Types. This is extremely powerful and can help take the guesswork out of the route back to true health and balance."

**—Shelley Riutta MSE,** founder and president of the Global
Association of Holistic Psychotherapy and Coaching

"Stress and how it affects the body is the number one topic while working with my clients. This book is a wealth of information. It delves deep into the biochemical effects of stress on our body—making it easy to understand—while providing solutions that don't feel overwhelming. I love it and plan on recommending it!"

**—Kiley Holmes, PT, DPT, OCS, SCS, FAAOMPT**

# MASTER YOUR STRESS, RESET YOUR HEALTH

The Personalized Program
to Calm Anxiety, Boost Energy,
and Beat Burnout

## DR. DONI WILSON

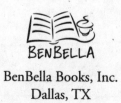

BenBella Books, Inc.
Dallas, TX

BenBella Books, Inc.
10440 N. Central Expressway
Suite 800
Dallas, TX 75231
benbellabooks.com
Send feedback to feedback@benbellabooks.com

*BenBella* is a federally registered trademark.

Printed in the United States of America
10 9 8 7 6 5 4 3 2 1

Library of Congress Control Number: 2021049864
ISBN 9781953295576 (print)
ISBN 9781953295910 (ebook)

Editing by Gregory Newton Brown and Claire Schulz
Copyediting by Jennifer Brett Greenstein
Proofreading by Michael Fedison
Indexing by WordCo Indexing Services
Text design and composition by PerfecType, Nashville, TN
Cover design by Emily Weigel
Printed by Lake Book Manufacturing

Special discounts for bulk sales are available. Please contact bulkorders@benbellabooks.com.

*To my patients, my daughter, and my parents for all you have taught me about being a human, in connection with others, exposed to stress, and being committed to living an inspired life. I dedicate this book to you.*

# Contents

CONTENTS

# PART III: THE THREE-PART STRESS RECOVERY PROTOCOL

# INTRODUCTION

# Healing the Burned-Out Body

A re you feeling uncomfortable in your body and overwhelmed in your life? You are in the right place. Likely you know what it's like to get caught up in "stress mode." The constant and pervasive sense of low-grade panic. The irritability. The fatigue. The frustration. The endless loops of self-criticism that tell us we always need to earn more, be more, do more, and succeed more.

Many of us have acknowledged with a certain amount of resignation that we are burned-out. We accept the physical signs—headaches, tension, brain fog, anxiety, and indigestion—as inevitable side effects of being a high achiever. We publicly wear "being so busy" as a badge of honor, while suffering silently and privately, afraid to look like the weak link who can't handle the demands of their job or life.

But what if I told you it's not that simple? My research and experience with patients have shown me that everyone has a unique stress type and a unique way to master their stress.

Do you have a compulsive need to be always on the go? Perhaps you've described yourself as having "high-functioning anxiety" because you feel pushed to work harder and longer. Do you feel persistent nervousness and also have frequent digestion issues? All of this means you might be what I call a Stress Magnet, a person plagued by consistently high cortisol throughout the day.

Or do you find that you're most productive late at night? Do you feel suddenly motivated to catch up on chores after 10 PM, pull all-nighters to finish projects you were too tired to work on during the day, or fall victim to late-night snacking and Netflix binges? You might be a Night Owl, a person whose adrenal imbalances peak in the evening, making them unable to "turn off."

Alternatively, you might not relate to either of those types because you never feel like you have much energy at all, regardless of the time of day. If you pretty much always feel tired, depressed, or generally unmotivated, you might be the Blah and Blue type, a person who wakes up with cortisol levels that start low and stay low, leaving them wanting to pull the blankets back over their head and disappear.

You may already feel like you recognize your stress type from these short descriptions, but once you do the self-assessment quiz included in this book, you'll be better able to identify your stress type. The types are important because treatment and management look different for every person. Think of it this way: your body is built to deal with stress—not just work stress, but also physical stress from your diet and from environmental toxins—and that means *it's also built to recover*. Just as a common cold won't kill you if your immune system is functioning optimally, stress won't turn into debilitating burnout if your recovery systems are functioning optimally.

By fine-tuning our built-in response to stress, we can learn to live with greater resiliency.

## How Stress Taught Me

I came to this understanding of stress through lived experience. For more than two decades, I lived with severe, debilitating migraines. Once or twice a month, I'd wake up with excruciating pain that quickly led to nausea and vomiting for hours on end. It took me days to recover. When this happened in naturopathic medical school, I still had to keep up, no matter how bad I felt. Later, as a mom and practicing naturopathic doctor, I found myself needing to reschedule patients and activities with my daughter so that I could lie in bed or on the bathroom floor for days at a time. I knew I had to find a better way.

I tried all sorts of diet changes and various systems of medicine—from acupuncture to massage therapy to detoxification to hormone balancing—and I found that solving my migraines came down to three steps.

First, I needed to accept my body for what it was. My genes and stress exposure set me up for migraines. I couldn't go get another body, but I could do something different with the one I had. Instead of rejecting my body and being mad at myself for something I couldn't change, I decided to embrace it.

Second, I needed to gather information. I looked at my genes and figured out how to support my body based on my genetics. I also looked at my stress exposure—including stress created by eating the wrong foods, being exposed to toxins, and shouldering expectations that I put on myself—and noticed where negative side effects occurred. I measured my cortisol and adrenaline levels and did a test to learn which bacteria were living in my gut so that I could correct what was out of balance.

Third, I had to choose differently. I discovered that I have a gene called *MTHFR* and that I require a certain quantity of the right B vitamins each day. Then, when I realized that I have a gene that causes my joints to be hyper-mobile, which means sitting in the same position for long periods of time is the worst possible thing for me, I ordered a standing desk and made sure to never sit for more than an hour at a time. When I tested my toxin levels and found that my body was filled with flame retardants from the mattress I slept on, I threw out that mattress and took nutrients to get rid of the toxins. After exploring the patterns on a deep emotional level, I realized that the migraines were my body's way of taking a break from my overly busy schedule. Once I made sure to plan more stress recovery in my schedule, my body didn't have to create a migraine in order for me to take time for myself.

Instead of giving up and giving in to a life of pain meds, I knew I had to do something to figure this out, and I did. As I made these gradual changes, my last headache soon went away. Then my anxiety about the next episode disappeared for good.

Migraines aren't the only signs of burnout that are now in my past. I don't have autoimmunity, even though my parents and grandparents did. I used to have allergies, sensitivities to many foods, fatigue, menstrual cramps, and depression. Now those issues are all gone, too.

It's been exciting to share this knowledge with my patients and watch them reap the benefits of equally impressive results. I've helped patients who previously had recurrent miscarriages finally achieve healthy pregnancies and healthy babies. I've helped women with abnormal pap smears rebalance their hormones and get back to healthy pap smears without procedures that could damage their cervix. I've helped men and women who no longer knew how they can get through another day due to fatigue, anxiety, insomnia, and/or pain live their passions and feel good doing it. I've helped adults and children who've been told that their immune systems are attacking their own bodies to reverse autoimmunity without the risks of immunosuppressive medications.

Stress, anxiety, and burnout manifest differently for everyone. So, how does your body signal burnout? Is it pain, fatigue, bloating, weight gain, anxiety, sleeplessness, infertility, infections, lack of muscle, low sex drive, or autoimmunity? Instead of brushing it under the rug or giving up, I'm going to teach you about a hidden factor that is causing you to feel awful. Perhaps you feel like you've tried everything, and nothing worked. That's because you haven't addressed adrenal distress. This book will show you that you have the power to give your body the support it needs to feel better, no matter how busy or stressed-out you are, and no matter how your distress manifests.

## Understanding Adrenal Distress

The problem for many of us today is chronic stress and subsequent adrenal distress, a condition marked by imbalances of the stress hormones adrenaline and cortisol, which hinder the body's natural ability to bounce back and recover after a stressful event; this results in burnout, anxiety, pain, and fatigue.

Healing from adrenal distress is as "simple" as correcting the imbalance. But since every person is different, what helps balance someone with overly high cortisol may be very detrimental for someone whose cortisol is chronically low. This is why making diet and lifestyle adjustments and taking supplements according to what I call your "stress type" are key.

It's also essential to implement stress recovery in a step-by-step fashion. If you were to skip step one, you could land yourself right back in stress mode again. It's through the process of helping patients recover from adrenal distress that I've developed my Stress Recovery Protocol. I'll be sharing it with you in this book, so you can have the information you need to recover most efficiently. It's well known that stressing about stress just makes things worse. Instead, I want you to de-stress in a systematic and strategic way that helps you achieve resilience to stress.

To do this successfully, you need to fully understand your built-in stress response system. I'll explain this system to you and guide you in mastering your ability to maintain health even while exposed to stress. A key aspect of achieving this is to realize that your body does not exist merely from the neck down. Throughout this book, when I use the term *body*, I'm referring to everything from the top of your head to the bottom of your feet, including your mind and your spirit.

## Sound Familiar?

During the last twenty-two years, I have treated thousands of men, women, and children who have come to me with a wide variety of symptoms—from fatigue, anxiety, depression, and pain to stomach ulcers, irritable bowel syndrome (IBS), heartburn, bloating, constipation, frequent or chronic infections, allergies, skin rashes, autoimmunity, thyroid conditions, menstrual-related symptoms, fertility issues, insomnia, and nervous system issues such as headaches or neuropathy. The most severe cases have involved conditions that can even develop into diabetes, cancer, and/or dementia. Patients come to me because they feel they've tried everything, without adequate results. Often, I've been told that, up until they met me, no health care provider mentioned that adrenal distress could be the true root of their illness.

These symptoms may sound wide-ranging, but they often come back to the same root cause: stress. My proven C.A.R.E. method of clean eating, adequate sleep, recovery, and exercise is effective in treating all these symptoms because it's designed to target that root cause. While I recommend that all my patients follow the C.A.R.E. method, each step of that program will mean something slightly different depending on their stress type.

Most of all, I can see that these recommendations are desperately needed. Our environments are becoming increasingly stressful due to a cultural trend toward chronic lack of sleep and excessive sugar consumption; the increased toxins in our air, water, and food; and the general prevalence of mold and pesticides. And that's before we even get to the psychological effects of a pandemic, social media, the expectation of 24/7 availability, and other adverse effects from demanding work and social environments influenced by mobile devices. All these triggers have negative effects on our bodies. They disrupt naturally robust biorhythms designed to regulate stress, making it harder for our bodies to function.

## How to Use This Book

In the first part of this book, you'll learn all about adrenal distress, including our built-in stress response system involving cortisol and adrenaline. You'll get a clear sense of how and why stress affects us, the types of stress we're potentially exposed to in our lifetimes, and how stress turns on our genetic susceptibilities. You'll also discover and reflect on the personal and cultural reasons why it's so hard to stay ahead of stress. And you'll see why mastering stress recovery is possible and life changing. By understanding stress and how it affects you, you'll be better able to make the necessary changes to recover from burnout and prevent it from happening again.

I'll guide you through a quiz to discover your stress type. You'll also consider other tests to help you see how stress has disrupted your health, not to mention what needs to be addressed to reset and recover from stress exposure. What's more, I'll teach you how to integrate C.A.R.E.—clean eating, adequate sleep, recovery, and exercise—into your unique schedule. Finally, I'll introduce you to the phases of the Stress Recovery Protocol, which will help you know where to start and which supplements (herbs and nutrients) best fit your stress type.

By the time you reach the final chapters, you'll be ready to maintain the stress recovery you have worked hard to achieve. Resilience to stress is ultimately the name of the game. I want you to have the knowledge and tools to bounce back from any stress that comes your way. And the ability to choose which challenges and stresses you'd like to invite into your life.

I don't want you to feel limited by stress or as if waves of stress are crashing over you and continually knocking you down throughout your day. Instead, I want you to be like a rock on the shoreline. You'll let the waves hit you, but you'll stand strong. Stress (wind, rain, waves) may erode a rock over thousands of years and shape it into something amazing—have you seen the Devil's Punch Bowl on the Oregon coast or the arch formations in Cabo San Lucas and Aruba? Rock formations exist around the world, demonstrating how nature responds to stress. Just as an irritant inside an oyster shell turns into a pearl, I want you to respond to stress, recover, and create the beautiful life of your dreams.

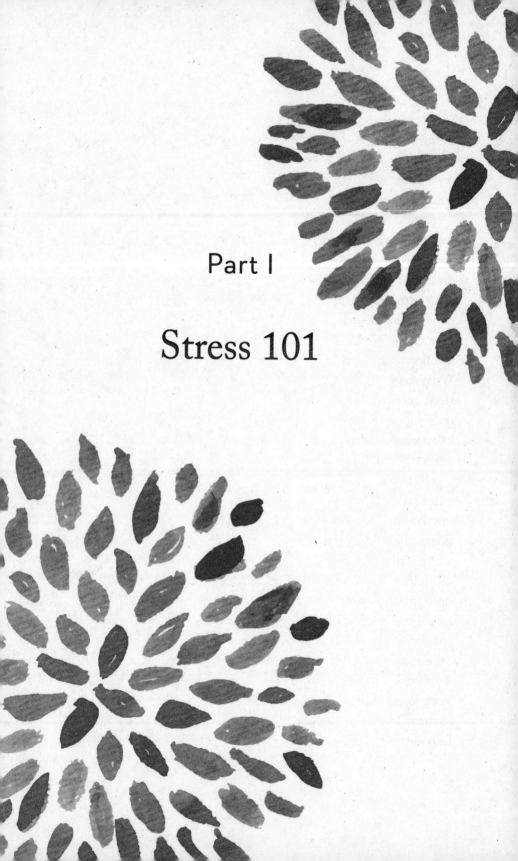

# Part I

# Stress 101

# What Happens When We're Stressed?

Nature versus nurture is a well-known, age-old debate about whether our personality, intelligence, and other traits are inherited (based on our genetics) or we acquire them through experiences and interactions. The phrase "nature versus nurture" was first documented by Sir Francis Galton, an English anthropologist, explorer, and founder of eugenics (now disproven) in the 1800s. The question essentially is whether genetics or environment has a more dominant influence over health. The answer, according to Galton, who looked to twins for the answer, was that genetics plays the stronger role in determining how our well-being unfolds. In fact, subsequent twin studies went on to demonstrate that genetics even plays a role in factors previously thought to be wholly determined by environment, like personality and mental illness.[1] (That said, it's important and also interesting to keep in mind that up until 1990 the studied twins all experienced a major stress in being ethically or unethically separated from each other and their parents at birth.)

Believing that genetics played an influential role in who we are and how our health evolved, doctors and scientists made a significant effort to map the human genes in our bodies with the hope of solving illness. Yet, when the thirteen-year-long international Human Genome Project was completed in 2003, they discovered that our health actually has less to do with our genes than previously thought! It blew everyone's mind to find out that genetics accounted for only up to 20 percent of the illnesses we experience. The major player, they found, in determining health issues is—drum roll, please—stress exposure.

At the same time, avoiding stress isn't the solution to our health problems. In fact, attempting to avoid stress actually causes more stress. Our stress response system is what helps us survive dangers and accomplish our goals. The solution is understanding and supporting the careful balance of stress and anti-stress.

## Understanding Epigenetics

When doctors realized that stress is a major player in health outcomes, swapping out a few genes to change one's fate was no longer a solution. While genetics plays a role in the tendency toward many health issues, stress is the factor that most influences whether a gene expresses itself in a way that affects our health.

The study of the influence of stress on genetic expression is called epigenetics. With epigenetic changes, stress (of various types) overrides the genetic message, turning genes on or off. Think of it this way: we are conceived and born with genetic tendencies that are dormant in quiet genes, and, depending on our stress exposure, may or may not be expressed. Depending on our various stress exposures, inherited tendencies can be more or less likely to present themselves.[2]

Epigenetics actually gives us the power to control our health more consciously than we ever realized. However, we need to learn how to manage stress exposure in a way that doesn't turn on our genetic tendencies, and to implement stress recovery that allows us to turn off our inherited health issues.

Isn't it amazing and empowering to know your health isn't set in stone? You have the ability to change your health every day of your life by understanding your genetic predispositions and by choosing to give your body what it needs to recover from stress.

Our internal and external environment (our stress exposure) can over-power our genetics. When our bodies think they are in a healthy environment (internal in particular), it shifts how genes are expressed.

How do we create a healthy internal environment, despite stress on the outside or in the past?

We do things and take supplements that shift cortisol and adrenaline in the direction they need to go in our bodies to get back to optimal, healthy levels. We heal the damage caused by stress. We heal leaky gut; balance our hormones, neurotransmitters, and gut bacteria; and get our immune systems back on track.

We essentially need to get *out* of stress mode and turn off our stress type, behaviors we'll learn later in the book with the C.A.R.E. method and my Stress Recovery Protocol.

## What's Stress Got to Do with It?

Despite the stress you're under, it's possible to take a deep breath, stand back, look around, and realize that we are the ones who *choose* to be the hamster on the hamster wheel.

As much as it may seem that you're destined to experience burnout based on the relationships, jobs, commitments, deadlines, and beliefs you hold in a modern, busy world, your current situation isn't your only option.

As you gain awareness, you'll see that you're repeating patterns that lead to an unhealthy body, mind, and spirit—and that, in fact, you can make deci-sions to change these. After all, you can change jobs, relationships, homes, food, routines, and even your sleep schedule. Heck, you can even change your religion or the country you live in if that makes a difference. It may seem impossible and improbable to do so, and usually such major changes are not necessary, but change in order to shift the patterns of stress in our lives isn't just possible—it's doable.

Inertia, on the other hand, is the tendency to remain unchanged. Unless forced to shift, we remain set on the path we are on. By understanding what has us stuck, we can figure out how to break free and make the changes that move us toward a healthier body and life.

When it comes down to it, most everything we do is a potential stress. Going to school, being a parent, running a business, having a job, being in a relationship, owning assets, and traveling are all examples of activities that are part of life and involve some amount of stress. In fact, we need stress hormones to signal our bodies to accomplish tasks. The type of stress we require to get things done is called eustress, and it is considered normal and even beneficial.

At times in human history, our lives have depended on our ability to respond under stress, and under sustained stress in particular. Think of how our ancestors navigated great migrations, crossing the ocean on a ship or riding on a covered wagon across the United States (which was the case for my ancestors). They didn't know what was coming next—whether they would have food and water, let alone a warm shelter and clothing. Their built-in stress responses helped them prepare for dangers and kept them focused on their goals. They kept them alive.

Bouts of stress like the ones I just described are what the body is equipped to experience. Long-term, recurrent stress, however, takes a negative toll on the body. In earlier times, our ancestors were likely to die from an infection, injury, or malnutrition before the age of sixty. Now, we are better able to prevent or treat those causes of death. However, we are exposed to much longer periods of stress, which can lead to heart disease, cancer, dementia, and other diseases and health conditions. With this awareness, researchers have studied centenarians (people who live to at least 100 years of age) in various cultures with hopes of discovering their secret to a long life. Over and over, these studies show that it comes down to both living in a way that allows for the most stress recovery and choosing to adapt to challenging life experiences.[3] Ruminating on a problem and having a closed or fixed mindset is associated with being less healthy. And yet, stress itself triggers ruminating thoughts, creating a cycle of more and more stress. We become stuck in the stress pattern, in what I call "stress mode," and even addicted to it.

What we need to change, then, is not only how we react to stress but our awareness of it and our willingness and ability to recover from it.

Stress without stress recovery has the potential to cause negative effects in our bodies, disrupting our ability to function in the most basic sense. For this reason, the best way to influence our health and risk for health issues is to understand the various types of stresses we are exposed to. That way, we can avoid excess stress whenever possible and provide ourselves with recovery practices. Instead of judging the stresses you experience or becoming fearful of possible future stresses, the way to break the pattern of stress is to come from a place of self-acceptance and acceptance of your life experiences. From there, consider how you could make choices to process and recover from those stress exposures.

So, why is it that in our modern society we allow ourselves to race through each day as though everything must be completed before we hit the pillow, when we know the health risks of stress? After all, feeling stressed has been shown to increase the risk of a heart attack by 27 percent, which is the same increase that occurs from smoking five cigarettes a day. And studies show that when people know about the effects of stress, they tend to stress about stress, compounding the situation![4]

What's just as bad is to ignore stress and power through. Acting invincible gets us nowhere. Even if we don't think we're stressed, we do still have a stress response and stress hormones. After all, we are not living in robot bodies. We are living in human bodies. By understanding the stress response and human need for stress recovery, we can stop being run by old patterns and change the effect that stress has on us.

The goal is to stop stressing about your stress responses, all while giving your body the support it needs to recover from the various stresses it faces. So many of us live in physical and emotional pain. We search long and hard for a magic pill or quick fix, when, really, the solution lies in understanding our stress response and recognizing how we can keep our bodies healthy while under stress.

At the heart of extreme stress and burnout is a term I've coined, "adrenal distress," which is ultimately the topic of this book. To really understand the stress and adrenal gland connection, you must understand our very human stress response, including how it *helps* us deal with stress. With understanding, which is a form of acceptance, you can begin to change the way that you think about stress and become curious about how your body in particular responds to it. In fact, what I'll be teaching you is that just as both genetics and stress exposure influence our health in general, they also both create our unique, individualized stress response.[5]

Let's look closer at stress responses and their unique patterns. Then we'll move into a deeper exploration of how chronic stress affects our bodies and how it's possible to support that system during both high and low periods of stress to avoid long-term ramifications.

## All About the Stress Response

Our human bodies are constantly perceiving potential stresses. Our eyes are looking for changes in our environment that could be dangerous and require a stress response. Our ears are listening for stress. Our noses are even smelling for potential stress. Ultimately, it's an almond-shaped part of the brain on each side of our head called the amygdala that receives a stress signal from our senses, recognizes the signals as a cause for fear, and alerts the rest of our body to danger.

First, the amygdala signals the part of our nervous system that responds without us thinking about it, called the autonomic nervous system (ANS). Day in and day out, the ANS sends messages within our bodies to make sure that we keep breathing and that our hearts keep beating, even while we sleep. It determines how much blood and oxygen to send to our muscles versus our digestive and reproductive organs, at any given time. There are two parts to the autonomic nervous system:

1. the sympathetic nervous system (SNS), which is responsible for the fight, flight, or freeze response
2. the parasympathetic nervous system (PNS), which is all about "rest and digest" and recovering from stress

When the amygdala picks up on stress, it tells the SNS to respond with adrenaline to help protect us from whatever perceived danger is at hand.

Next, the amygdala sends a message to the hypothalamus in the brain, which makes a hormone called corticotropin-releasing hormone (CRH). This hormone signals the pituitary gland (also in the brain) to make a hormone called adrenocorticotropic hormone (ACTH). Blood transports ACTH to the adrenal glands, which are above the kidneys, prompting them to release two stress hormones, adrenaline (more of it) and cortisol, into the blood. This stress response pathway from the brain to the adrenals is referred to as the hypothalamic-pituitary-adrenal axis (HPA axis). As the cortisol level in the blood increases, the hypothalamus picks up on the rising level and turns off the stress message.[6] Essentially, the adrenal stress response signals back to the brain that the stress has been managed and the CRH and ACTH should be turned off, or turned down.

This ability of our bodies to come back to balance is referred to as homeostasis. Actually, our bodies thrive on homeostasis. It allows us to have a little "wiggle room" in our state of being. We can exercise, increase our activity, or essentially challenge ourselves a bit, increasing our stress level somewhat, without totally throwing our bodies off track, because our bodies have a corrective response that will bring us back in balance. I think of it like a carriage return on an old-style typewriter (yes, that's how I learned to type). We can stray away, to some degree, from our set point, which is slightly different for each person, and then our internal systems know how to bring us back to that set point. Let's look more closely at how that process works.

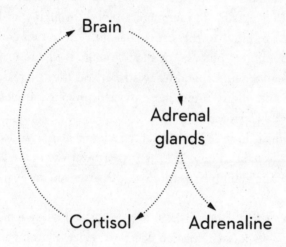

Brain

Adrenal glands

Cortisol        Adrenaline

## Sending Out an SOS

When stress comes along, whether emotional or physical, it kicks off an adrenaline rush that happens so quickly, you might not even realize that there's stress happening to even respond to. Meanwhile, your body will already have its fight-or-flight response in high gear. That's why you'll hear about people responding or acting at the scene of a car accident before even thinking about what's happening. When you think about it, every part of the stress response system has a specific purpose that helps us respond to stresses and survive. Even the "freeze" response is important for helping us prepare to protect ourselves. Let's look at the stress response system in a bit more detail and understand how each of the signals and hormones along the way plays a role in helping us respond to stress.

When we discuss stress hormones, we often talk about two main players, cortisol and adrenaline. (We'll get to cortisol in a minute.) Actually, what we call "adrenaline" is itself two different but related substances: epinephrine (adrenaline) and norepinephrine (noradrenaline); together, they're known as catecholamines. Norepinephrine is released by the sympathetic nervous system, and both norepinephrine and epinephrine are released into the bloodstream by the adrenal glands, specifically from a part of the gland called the adrenal medulla. Norepinephrine and epinephrine increase heart contractions and heart rate, while simultaneously increasing blood pressure; this makes it possible to pump more blood through your body faster, so that you can respond to the stress at hand. These two chemicals also increase the amount of glucose, or blood sugar, available in your blood, which you'll need when responding to stress, and they increase both your breathing rate and ability to get more oxygen to your muscles and brain, increasing mental alertness.[7]

Cortisol is made in the outer layer of the adrenal glands, called the cortex. Cortisol joins adrenaline in an effort to increase glucose in the bloodstream, enhancing the brain's ability to use glucose; this gives you the energy and focus to respond.

Meanwhile, cortisol decreases other, less essential systems during an immediate stress response. Digestion decreases, since digesting food is less of a priority when your body is responding to stress. Hormone production also decreases, including hormones made by the ovaries, testes, and thyroid glands. Immune system function generally decreases during the stress response, although for some people the immune system shifts into an overactive pattern. The nervous system pumps out stimulating neurotransmitters and uses up calming neurotransmitters all at the same time.

Our stress response system includes a shut-off mechanism as well, referred to as negative feedback. Receptors in the hypothalamus notice the cortisol level increasing and subsequently turn off the stress signal to the HPA axis. As soon as the stress response turns off, things go back to usual. Adrenaline and cortisol shift to optimal levels (not zero) for daily functioning. The autonomic nervous system shifts from sympathetic to parasympathetic. Breathing slows, as does the heart. Digestive function and hormone production return to optimal. The immune system goes back to protecting you from foreign invaders, and the nervous system calms down.

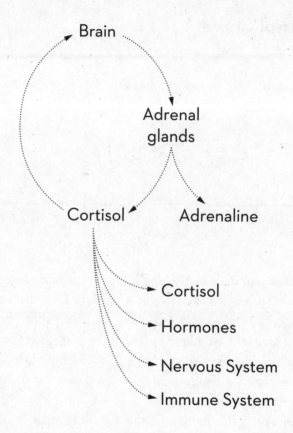

## Understanding Cortisol and Neurotransmitters

Mastering stress is about having an optimal amount of cortisol and adrenaline. Let's take a minute to learn more about the fascinating hormone called cortisol.

Cortisol levels vary with our circadian rhythm. Circadian rhythm is how our bodily functions align with the wake and sleep cycle (day and night) that comes with living on planet Earth. Cortisol levels rise in the early morning, coinciding with when you wake and giving you energy to start your day. There's an additional increase in cortisol within thirty to forty-five minutes after you wake called the cortisol awakening response (CAR), resulting in a 50 percent increase in cortisol levels. From there, the cortisol level gradually decreases throughout the day until it reaches its lowest at night, while you are sleeping.

## Cortisol Curve

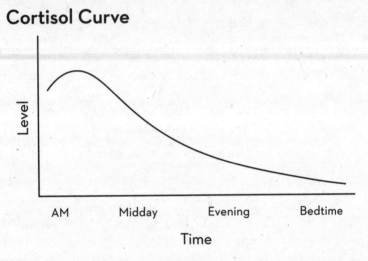

Interestingly, your daily cortisol levels follow a pattern unique to you. We now know there are genes related to cortisol and the CAR that influence how your body responds to waking up and to stress exposure throughout your life. Your body's response is as unique as your fingerprints. Even when you are exposed to an immediate stress, your body will come back to its daily cortisol levels. And those levels will influence how you feel each day and the quality of your health over time.

Let's consider this in a bit more detail. Cortisol signals to all other areas of the body, all the time. In this way, it acts like a central manager for our bodies. Cortisol communicates with the immune system, the digestive system, the nervous system, and the endocrine system—including all hormones, such as thyroid and insulin. These communications are essential for an effective stress response, but also for orchestrating all our daily functions and activities.

Cortisol is stimulating, so when it increases in the morning and wakes you up, it also signals to your nervous system to make neurotransmitters, which are messengers in the nervous system that help you focus, think, and solve problems—these neurotransmitters include serotonin, dopamine, norepinephrine, and epinephrine. These brilliant messengers set the speed of your brain and thinking. If your stress exposure is a bit high, this may cause dopamine to be higher, which can create rapid-fire thoughts and be helpful when you're dealing with an urgent challenge, but not so helpful if you need to focus on a single task.

Neurotransmitters also influence our mood, energy, and sleep. Ultimately, it's best to have a balance of stimulating and calming neurotransmitters. While dopamine and adrenaline are stimulating, serotonin and gamma aminobutyric acid (GABA) are calming. I think of GABA as our "stress buffer," because it can literally act like a shock absorber as we travel along the bumpy, stress-laden road of our lives.

For a long time, it was thought that the nervous system and neurotransmitters were untouchable due to a cellular wall called the blood-brain barrier (BBB), which was said to separate our nervous system from the rest of the body. We now know, however, that the brain and neurotransmitters are in full communication with the rest of our bodies and they are influenced by what we eat, by stress exposure, and by the bacteria (and other microbes) living in our intestines. In fact, all our neurotransmitters are made from amino acids, which come from the protein in our diet. At least 90 percent of serotonin is produced in the intestines, not our brain. This means we can influence our neurotransmitter levels, as well as mood, energy, focus, and sleep, through diet, nutrients, digestive health, and stress recovery.[8] The internal communication and interrelationship within our bodies is referred to as the gut-brain axis or gut-brain-microbiota axis, and it's the reason why I think of the mind and body not as separate entities but rather as a fully integrated system. Our bodies include our minds and spirits. By thinking of ourselves as separate parts functioning independently, we create more stress and block our ability to understand ourselves deeply as whole beings.

## CORTISOL EFFECTS

Cortisol signals to hormones throughout our bodies, including insulin. If cortisol and glucose remain high, our cells can become less responsive to insulin; this then leads to high blood sugar levels and what is referred to as metabolic syndrome or prediabetes, and eventually diabetes. Metabolism is how our bodies turn our food into energy. Our metabolic rate—how much energy we use on a daily basis—is affected by cortisol and adrenaline and influences our body weight.

Cortisol also affects the thyroid gland. The thyroid makes thyroid hormone, T4, which is converted to the active thyroid hormone, T3. T3 is stimulating, as it gives us energy to move around and get things done. It increases metabolism of nutrients into calories, which our muscles can burn as fuel. T3 signals throughout the body, affecting everything from mood and digestion to skin and energy. When cortisol levels shift higher or lower, the production of T4 and its conversion to T3 slow down. This can result in symptoms of low thyroid activity, such as fatigue, weight gain, hair loss, dry skin, and constipation.

What's more, the ovaries in women and testes in men are also influenced by cortisol, and their function decreases when cortisol is either too high or too low. This can affect estrogen, progesterone, and testosterone production, and increase or decrease fertility by influencing ovulation and sperm production. The body knows that times of stress aren't optimal for reproduction. In addition to affecting fertility in both sexes, high or low cortisol levels can cause women to experience missed periods, low libido, irregular menstrual cycles, premenstrual symptoms, cramping, and even early menopause. For men, they can result in low libido and fatigue.

Cortisol communicates with the digestion system, as well. Think of this interplay as a balancing act or tightrope walk. When just the right amount of cortisol is present, your digestive system is ready to receive food, digest it, and allow nutrients to be absorbed into your body through the cells lining the intestinal walls. At the same time, the liver is processing toxins and making bile, which enters the intestines via the gallbladder. Fiber and waste exit your body in feces, and every part of this process requires consistent signaling from cortisol. At any point along the way, if a stress signal turns off the digestion, you won't digest your food or absorb the nutrients from your food as well as you should. The intestinal cells become less healthy, leading to intestinal permeability (also known as leaky gut), and allow undigested food to leak through the intestinal walls where it triggers an inflammatory response. The healthy bacteria living in your intestines are disrupted, and your bowels may not move as consistently as when you are calm.[9]

It's also possible that the originating stress signal came from your digestion, perhaps from a food triggering an inflammatory response or undesirable bacteria releasing a toxin. A signal is sent from the intestines to the brain, via cortisol and the vagus nerve, telling it to shut down normal digestive function in order to address the stress. This pathway is referred to as the gut-brain axis, and it can lead to a vicious cycle of stress and digestive issues. It is so important that we'll cover it in more detail later.

Essentially, any slight variation in cortisol levels from minute to minute, hour to hour, or day to day can shift the signaling to your digestion and your ability to get nutrients from your food. It also shifts the function of your immune system. You see, the immune system works on a continuum and involves many different types of cells and signaling molecules/substances. When completely in balance and on track, your immune system is ready to protect you from anything it deems as foreign, such as viruses, bacteria, and parasites. When it is askew due to stress exposure and cortisol levels that are higher or lower than your "usual," your immune system becomes less able to fend off infections. At the same time, you are more likely to experience allergies or even autoimmunity, which occurs when the immune system attacks your own healthy cells. This is because stress dysregulates the immune system, making you vulnerable to viruses that can trigger autoimmunity, and it turns on your genetic predispositions to autoimmunity.

While cortisol is essential for functioning each day and we need it as part of our life-preserving response to stress at a second's notice, keeping ourselves in a constant stress response leads to cortisol levels that are not optimal in the long term. Digestive issues begin to develop, along with imbalanced hormones, depleted neurotransmitters, and less optimal immune function. It is well established that stress and cortisol levels outside the optimal range are responsible for triggering various health issues, including anxiety; depression; insomnia; fatigue; brain fog; weight gain; fertility issues; low thyroid function; diabetes; digestive disturbances such as irritable bowel syndrome (IBS), ulcers, and bloating; and immune-related issues like frequent infections, allergies, acne and eczema, autoimmunity, and cancer.

## Mind and Body Are One

Let's stop for a second. I want to further dissolve the concept that your mind and body are two separate entities. They aren't! They are one interconnected system. We always hear about our "mental health" and "physical health" or "mind and body," but I want to encourage you to shift that thinking.

Additionally, we tend to think of top-down communication as that which occurs from the brain down throughout the body. And, in fact, the major parts of the stress response we've been discussing, the HPA axis and autonomic nervous system, do function in that manner. However, it's important to recognize that communication also occurs in the opposite direction, from the bottom up, so to speak. Stress and anti-stress signals from within the body travel up to the brain, as well.

The gut-brain axis is a perfect example of how the mind and body are completely interconnected and how communication travels in both directions. The vagus nerve is the main part of the parasympathetic nervous system and is known as the longest nerve in the body, stretching from the brain down to the digestion system.[10] It is essentially a superhighway, containing over one hundred thousand nerve fibers, with signals going back and forth with vital information. It is a key element of the gut-brain connection and is special because the brain sends information to the gut and, in return, the gut can send information back to the brain. That is why the gut is considered the second brain and is a regulator of so many functions in the body.

The more your brain perceives stress, the more it affects your gut. The more your gut is stressed, the fewer enzymes it produces, the less able it is to digest your food, the fewer nutrients you absorb, the more the gut bacteria become imbalanced, the more severe leaky gut, and the more stress is communicated back to your nervous system. It's all related! There is no way to determine what came first, the brain or the body, so to speak. It's like the "chicken and the egg" debate. Patients sometimes ask me, "Is it possible that my gut is related to health in other areas of my body?" when they have increasing health issues that they just can't figure out. My response is always "Yes! It's all happening in your one human body, so it is most definitely all related. It's not a long list of issues, but one issue that is showing up in many ways."

The same is true for the heart-brain connection. From an anatomical and physiological perspective, we think of our hearts as pumping blood throughout our bodies and returning it to our lungs to get more oxygen. At the same time, when we think of a heart shape, or send a heart emoji, we are thinking of the emotion of love. But it turns out that our anatomical hearts are involved in communicating emotions and stress to our brains and vice versa, also via the vagus nerve. Think of how your heart races when you feel excited or stressed. Knowing this, you can choose activities that purposely send calming signals along these pathways. These same activities can increase the hormone oxytocin, the love hormone, which slows the heart rate and protects your heart from stress. As your heart rate decreases, so does your stress response. You can actually measure your heart rate to monitor this effect, too (more on that in chapter eight).

By understanding the autonomic nervous system and the vagus nerve, we begin to see how interconnected our bodies are. Not only that, but we can also see how they correlate to the ancient system from India of understanding the human energy centers, known as chakras. The seven main chakras are the root, sacral, solar plexus, heart, throat, third eye, and crown, corresponding with the major nerve networks and glands producing hormones in our bodies. We need them to be in sync and flowing in order to feel well.

## Understanding Adrenaline

Now, let's take a good look at adrenaline. Adrenaline doesn't fluctuate with the circadian rhythm the way cortisol does. It is pretty steady throughout the day and night, unless, of course, your stress response is triggered, in which case it spikes and then returns to a baseline level.

Adrenaline is active in the nervous system, acting as a neurotransmitter that stimulates activity, thoughts, and actions. Adrenaline, as we've discussed, also acts throughout the body on the blood vessels, heart, and muscles to get you moving and responding. You need it for daily activities, exercise, thinking, moving, and even breathing. You wouldn't want to live without adrenaline, yet when there is too much or too little at any given time, it can make you feel like you are completely out of sync.

The neurotransmitter dopamine converts to norepinephrine and then epinephrine. Next, norepinephrine and epinephrine are processed further to small molecules called metabolites, which can be eliminated in your urine. The process is essentially a cascade within your cells, converting one substance to the next. This cascade requires certain nutrients, including magnesium and B vitamins, and is genetically unique. Some of us process adrenaline more quickly and are more likely to become depleted. Others process adrenaline slowly, and while they can still become depleted, more often their adrenaline levels will remain higher than optimal way after the stress has cleared.

Knowing your adrenaline level and how your body handles it is critical for stress recovery. In fact, later in the book, I'll guide you to address high adrenaline first, before addressing low cortisol. High adrenaline tells you that you're in stress mode. If it continues, it won't matter what else you do, because stress mode will be working against you. It's essential to help your body get out of stress mode and get adrenaline back to a healthy level to give yourself the best chance of creating resilience to stress.

## Stress Resilience

Scientists use the term *hormesis* to describe a situation in which a small amount of a substance or change (a stress) is beneficial, but a large amount has a negative effect.[11] In small doses (which are slightly different for each person), these stressors shift you away from homeostasis just enough to induce an adaptive positive effect.

With hormesis, pathways within the body signal cellular repair, a process called autophagy, where cells clean out dysfunctional proteins and unnecessary debris.[12] A burst of oxidative stress—caused by free radicals disrupting healthy molecules—turns on the production of glutathione, a major antioxidant produced in our bodies, allowing for the repair of DNA. Plus there is an increase in the number of new mitochondria (the energy-producing organelles inside our cells), improved elimination of toxins, reduced inflammation, and enhanced resiliency to other stresses.

It is now believed that exposure to hormetic stressors can prevent health issues, including cancer and dementia, and improves longevity.[13] Examples of activities that trigger hormesis (which I'll discuss in more detail later in the book) are exercise, intermittent fasting, and cold exposure. It's tempting to think that more is better; however, I want to warn you that hormesis is dose dependent and unique to each individual based on your current state of stress.

## You Are Human

Developing awareness of and resilience to stress is one thing. But it's another thing to believe that you're a superhuman performer who can withstand stress at all costs. I warn patients that this way of thinking simply delays the inevitable point at which their body will collapse under the pressure of too much stress. This may present as a heart attack out of nowhere, or intractable insomnia after years of pushing through unrelenting stress, or exhaustion and lightheadedness that make it hard to get through the day.

It's true that, based on studies, stressing about stress doesn't help any situation.[14] But ignoring the fact that you are living in a human body that responds to stress is also just as harmful. Only by accepting the ways your body responds to stress as real and natural, and then understanding that the symptoms you experience are actually signals from within to make changes, can you realize that your stress response has become dramatically out of balance. Only then, after gaining the clarity of sight needed to heal, can you learn how to harness stress to empower yourself.

Getting out of stress mode, adjusting your choices and priorities, and feeling great start with understanding how you got into stress mode in the first place. Let's look at the physical signs that can alert you that your stress response system has gotten out of balance. After all, you can't start supporting your body better until you know how to see and hear your body's cry for help, right?

# What Is Adrenal Distress?

I t can be hard to imagine that emotional or psychological upsets like child-hood trauma, an unsupportive marriage or relationship, or a dead-end job in which you feel trapped could lead to physical health issues, but the medical community knows this to be true. When your life is besieged by long-term anxieties, your body begins to break down under stress, sometimes gradually and other times all at once. The end result is a laundry list of symptoms and diagnoses that require you to rein in your stress exposure in order to heal.

There are numerous long-term health issues linked to adrenal distress. These include but aren't limited to digestion issues (stomach ulcers, irritable bowel syndrome, inflammatory bowel disease, heartburn, bloating, consti-pation, diarrhea); immune-related conditions (autoimmunity, frequent infec-tions, acne, allergies, inflammation); nervous system problems (headaches, anxiety, depression, insomnia, neuropathy, attention issues, memory issues); and hormone-related concerns (thyroid issues, diabetes, weight gain, infertil-ity, low libido).[1] Stress is also linked to heart disease, cancer, dementia, and many other health conditions including accelerated aging.

If you're suffering from any of these illnesses, it's worth assessing whether stress might be responsible for your symptoms, especially if you've tried other types of treatment without success. The reason you haven't been able to solve the pain and suffering you are experiencing is because the real problem is hidden. As a naturopathic doctor, instead of going straight to prescription medications, I'm always looking for the root cause, and yet in the case of adrenal distress, the real cause of fatigue, anxiety, brain fog, weight gain, and joint pain is so buried, most practitioners miss it. This hidden factor also shows up differently in each person. We need to understand how your body uniquely responds to stress in order to know how to support you in your optimal stress pattern. At the same time, I want to help you shift the way you view what's happening in your body from "this is happening to me" to "symptoms are signals from my body telling me that it's overstressed and needs help to recover."

In this chapter, we'll discuss how to embrace stress as part of being human, how various stressors and genetic influences lead to adrenal distress, and how to become empowered by your ability to reverse the effects of stress on *your* health.

## Stress Without Enough Recovery

Stress, which comes in many different forms, is your body's way of responding to *any* kind of demand or change. The most common stress events are circumstantial: a death, a divorce, a new job, or a move to a new home. But there are also many physiological stressors that we overlook or push aside, such as not getting enough sleep, eating too much sugar, exposing our body to inflammatory foods, or even exposing it to toxins in our environment or personal care products.

The bottom line is that we are all exposed to stress, including stress from our childhood. I remember my mom telling me "Your dad is stressed!" when he'd come home from work feeling irritable. And she told me I was stressed when I came down with a sinus infection and slept for a week after finals in college.

It wasn't until years later that I really began to understand the effects of stress. While training to be a doula and a midwife, I studied women with a history of sexual abuse and how they experienced labor. Nearly all women experience fear when it comes to delivering a baby, but for women who have been through trauma, it's amplified.

What I found most interesting about working with women during this time is that our stress hormones—specifically, cortisol and adrenaline—are actually *necessary* for labor to progress effectively.[2] They signal to the uterus to contract and for the normal labor process to occur. When there is too much stress, such as when women (with or without a history of abuse) don't have enough support, labor comes to a complete standstill. However, labor also stops if there isn't enough cortisol and adrenaline. That's when Mother Nature's contradiction struck me most—the irony being that in order to properly harness stress, we need an equal or appropriate amount of *support* to balance that stress. How much we need is unique for each person.

I realized that what is observed in labor is true for daily life—we need an optimal amount of cortisol, adrenaline, and support for our bodies to perform at their best. If we don't get support to recover from stress, adrenal distress happens.

## What Does Adrenal Distress Look Like?

You may be familiar with what it feels like to be angling toward burnout, or what I call stress mode. It looks different for each of us. You may notice your mind races, your hands sweat, your heart beats fast, and you might feel a little (or very) nauseated—basically, the world seems like it's spinning out of control, and all you want to do is break the maddening cycle and return to normalcy. It can feel like there's too much to do and not enough time—as if everything in your life needs to be addressed immediately, yet there aren't enough minutes in the day for that to occur. After all, the project must be completed, and the house has to get cleaned, and the laundry must get done. A parent, child, friend, or loved one needs your help, *right now*. Your health issues may even have swept you into such a frenzy of trying to solve them that the stress of the health issue is creating more stress! Sleep, if you can get it, doesn't help you feel better. Cooking meals and sitting down to enjoy them has fallen by the wayside.

By the time you work your way through your endless list of urgent tasks each day, you are often too exhausted to think straight or enjoy a moment of calm.

Feeling this way isn't a sign that your body needs another cup of coffee or even a quick-fix nap. It's an indicator that you're experiencing disrupted adrenaline and cortisol levels, which means that your adrenal glands could use an assist before they crash and burn.

## Enter Adrenal Distress

Here's what all of this means in your day-to-day life: when you encounter a stress response, say an alarm suddenly going off at 6 AM, the cortisol and adrenaline rush is meant to give you the energy to remove yourself from the perceived danger—in this case, a sudden and alarming noise. A healthy body reacts to this perceived danger with spiking adrenaline and cortisol, which normalize when the stress trigger is gone.

You encounter a major issue when the "coming back down" doesn't happen. When you are under stress, day in and day out, without a break, the SNS and the HPA axis continually signal the production of adrenaline and cortisol. The hypothalamus stops turning off the stress signal because the receptors become desensitized. At the same time, the autonomic nervous system doesn't switch over to the PNS. Instead, it stays in fight-or-flight mode, pushing out large amounts of adrenaline. Even once the stress stops—say, the weekend comes, the deadline is over, the crisis has passed—the message of stress keeps on going inside your body. It's like the body gets stuck in stress mode.

Essentially, with long-term, repetitive stress exposure, your normal on-and-off switch for stress stops working correctly. Your body anticipates stress, constantly. You might feel the symptoms of stress all day or any time of day or night—whether your actual stress exposure is high or not. You might find your heart racing or palpitating, your blood pressure rising, or your mind racing, and then think to yourself, "What's going on? I feel stressed, but there's no stress in sight."

When you are stuck in stress mode, your adrenal glands will respond by making more cortisol and/or adrenaline, or they might not be able to keep up with the demand for those stress messengers. Depending on your genetics and how your body processes cortisol and adrenaline, as well as your personal and family history of stress exposure, your hormone output may lag or plummet. At that point, even when an actual stress does happen, your adrenals might be too overtaxed to produce adequately.

This is what I refer to as adrenal distress.

This doesn't mean that your adrenals have necessarily stopped working alto-gether and forever. The adrenal glands can recover from adrenal distress with the right care and attention—mainly, recognition of the problem and recovery time. Depending on whether your cortisol and/or adrenaline shift higher or lower, a potentially different set of symptoms can occur. You may experience fatigue, anxiety or a low mood, a foggy brain, and difficulty feeling motivated. It's important to note that this can happen at any age and isn't based on accu-mulated stress over time. Whether it happens, and when, is unique for each individual based on genetics and exposure to both stress and stress recovery.

While I treat adrenal distress (referred to as adrenal fatigue by some) all the time in my practice, I want to specifically state that it isn't well recog-nized in conventional medicine. Although it's referred to in studies as adrenal maladaptation syndrome and has been studied by physiologists for more than sixty years, starting with Dr. Hans Selye, it's not a diagnosis you're likely to receive from your internist or endocrinologist, like Addison's disease, in which the adrenals stop making cortisol altogether, or Cushing's disease, in which the level of cortisol skyrockets and doesn't come down, often due to medica-tions or a tumor.[3]

Imagine a light switch that has been flipped on so many times that it has become stuck in the on position. That's what leads to adrenal distress. But the switch can turn off again, I promise. Just as your body got into stress mode, it can get back out again. After all, if it can turn on your stress response, it can turn it off, too. Your body needs consistent anti-stress signals and various sup-ports to help your hypothalamus and adrenal glands to recover and respond appropriately again, bringing your digestion, hormones, immune system, and nervous system back online.

It's important to know, however, that it's not as simple as meditating on a rock. We have to approach your stress recovery from the perspective of your stress type. It's not one size fits all. Furthermore, once you have consistently appropriate levels of cortisol and adrenaline at the ready to respond to your optimal amount of stress, you will be more resilient to stress in general.

## A Closer Look at Adrenal Distress

As I mentioned in chapter one, cortisol should be higher in the morning and gradually decrease throughout the day. This hormone communicates with various other systems in our bodies, including the digestive system, immune system, nervous system, and endocrine (or hormone) system.

If you were to compare your body to a business, cortisol would be the supervising manager. It sends out signals to the rest of your body to say where to focus and what to do or not do. If not for cortisol, your body systems would be in complete chaos, like an orchestra without a director. Instruments would be playing whatever they chose, and whenever.

As cortisol shifts higher or lower, at different times of day or night, the other systems in your body follow. Higher than usual cortisol production for a particular time of day signals to turn off digestion, turn down hormone production, and shift the nervous and immune systems to stress response mode. It orchestrates a stress response throughout the body, which is fine and good for a short-term stressor. The problem occurs when the stress doesn't end and your cortisol level never has a chance to reset, as mentioned above. It would be as if a symphony crescendoed to forte, the loudest part of the song, and stayed there. Or as if a business manager assigned one deadline after the next, without giving the staff a chance to regroup and reorder supplies in between.

While your body can handle stress, things start to fall apart. There's no chance for you to digest food and move your bowels, or for your hormones to perform optimally. Stomach acid can cause burning in your stomach, due to a lack of protective mucus. Undigested food overfeeds bacteria leading to gas and bloating. Intestinal cells are not replaced fast enough, causing leaky gut, which sends inflammation throughout your body. Blood sugar levels fluctuate from high to low. Your body shifts to storing fat instead of burning fat. Hunger and fullness signals disappear or food cravings soar. Your libido goes kaput and (in women) your menstrual cycle goes haywire. Your immune system is pushed toward allergies, infections, and autoimmunity instead of maintaining a protective guard against the most important invaders. Your nervous system spins itself into a frenzy of excitotoxic glutamate and phenylalanine (PEA), which are stimulating neurotransmitters, in an attempt to respond to the stress signal, but ultimately damages your nerve cells in the process. And all those calming neurotransmitters that we talked about in the last chapter, including serotonin and GABA, become depleted as they work to buffer your stress. Brain fog sets in, as does pain and exhaustion.

What starts out as a healthy stress response becomes a nightmare of compounding. While you might experience everything mentioned in the last paragraph, and more, it's quite likely that you'll experience some symptoms more than others, depending on your susceptibilities as well as how your cortisol and adrenaline respond to stress. Your body is trying to tell you it needs help. The fatigue, anxiety, stomach troubles, sleep issues, and brain fog all start to become a message from your body that it's overstressed. At first, it may seem like a whisper. Little by little, as you understand how your body responds to stress, it will become clear that your body isn't doing this "to you." Stress is doing it to you, and it's up to you to show up to help your body.

The way your cortisol responds to stress is to some degree affected by your cortisol-related genes.[4] If you have genes that cause you to make more cortisol and faster, versus genes that make it more likely that you'll become depleted in cortisol, this will make a big difference in the way you feel, especially when you're stressed. We also know that if your ancestors were exposed to more stress, and/or if you were exposed to a high amount of stress in your childhood, you have a tendency to have higher cortisol. It all comes down to genes and enzyme pathways that determine whether cortisol is turned into an active form or remains in an anti-inflammatory form (cortisone).

At the same time, it's important to remember that adrenaline levels throw another variable into the mix. Adrenaline can be higher than desired when your body is stuck in a stress response. It's as if you're stepping on the gas pedal, whether you're ready to speed up or not. Now the orchestra is playing not only way too loud, but also far too quickly, under the influence of elevated adrenaline. Remember, adrenaline, otherwise known as norepinephrine and epinephrine, is made from dopamine, which comes from phenylalanine (PEA). Together, they are referred to as catecholamines, and they push the various systems of our body to respond and speed up in a stressful situation. If, while converting to dopamine and adrenaline, PEA gets stuck along the way, these catecholamines are more likely to build up. When this happens, the heart races, sweat pours, and the mind bounces from one thought to the next like a Mexican jumping bean. People with high levels of PEA and/or dopamine feel like *everyone else* is moving too slowly.

## GENETIC INFLUENCE

The ability of your catecholamines to convert PEA to dopamine, dopamine to norepinephrine, and norepinephrine to epinephrine is influenced by your stress and your genes. There are enzymes in your cells whose job is to make a chemical change to each substance in the sequence. These enzymes require nutrients, such as magnesium, iron, vitamin C, and S-adenosylmethionine (SAM), which is made from our B vitamins, and they are slowed down by various kinds of stress. Toxins on nonorganic food (pesticides), in water, and in the air (mold toxins), as well as toxins produced by unhealthy gut bacteria (known as lipopolysaccharides [LPS]), slow down the processing of catecholamines, which tends to lead to an increase in PEA, dopamine, and/or adrenaline.

Furthermore, having genetic variations on the genes that signal the production of these enzymes will influence the speed at which the enzymes work. What does all of this mean for you? If your enzymes are working too slowly, then you're more likely to have a buildup of adrenaline. If your enzymes are working too quickly, then you're more likely to become depleted in adrenaline. Both situations are an issue. High adrenaline will cause you to feel anxious and stressed all the time. Low adrenaline will cause you to feel tired and have brain fog.

The main enzyme involved in processing adrenaline (catecholamines) is catechol-O-methyltransferase (COMT). There are two variants of the *COMT* gene. Those who have the variant that breaks down adrenaline more quickly are referred to as having a "warrior gene" because when they're stressed, their adrenaline increases, helping them to respond, and then quickly returns to a non-stressed state so they can recover. Those with the other variant, referred to as the "worrier gene," break down catecholamines more slowly. When stressed, they are likely to have higher adrenaline for longer, which causes them to feel wired, overwhelmed, and irritable—sometimes even when it's time to relax. These effects are amplified in women because estrogen is also processed through COMT, causing a traffic jam and an additional increase in dopamine and adrenaline. People with either variant can learn ways to get the most out of their *COMT* genes, once they know that warriors may need a bit of stress to feel motivated and worriers may need a gradual introduction to new tasks in order to moderate their adrenaline levels.

Monoamine oxidase (MAO-A) is the enzyme that processes both adrenaline (catecholamines) and serotonin, one of our calming neurotransmitters. People who have a SNP, a single nucleotide polymorphism or gene variation (or two), of *MAO-A*, another warrior gene, tend to have lower serotonin and higher adrenaline because the *MAO* SNP speeds up the processing of serotonin while slowing down the elimination of adrenaline. When people have both *COMT* and *MAO* SNPs, they feel like they are driving a race car with super-tight steering and tight shocks. They're likely to feel every bump in the road, meaning that their nervous system is likely to give them signals for each and every stress, and they'll feel it more than others do. This can cause anxiety, irritability, and symptoms potentially diagnosed as attention deficit hyperactivity disorder (ADHD), bipolar disorder, and depression.[5] At the same time, it makes them good at surviving under stress. No matter what gene variations you have, the tools in this book will help you learn what your body needs to break up metabolic traffic jams and prevent severe pendulum swings in your energy and mood.

In the process of learning about gene variations and how they influence the way we feel, as well as what we can do to address them, what I kept hearing and reading over and over is that the best approach is to take steps to reduce stress exposure and then to support stress recovery. This is true because stress of various types—from emotional, to physical, to toxins from the environment and from imbalanced gut bacteria—all slow down or speed up our metabolic pathways. This means that on top of genetically determined variations, our stress exposure makes it all worse—it amplifies metabolic dysfunction. I think of it like a sink with a clogged drain. If the drain is clogged with stress, it won't matter whether we turn on the faucet and take more of a precursor nutrient, because instead of flowing through the metabolic process, the extra nutrient will just get stuck in the drain (so to speak) or the sink will overflow. We first need to clear out the drain by making diet changes, getting better sleep, recovering from stress, and exercising—exactly what is in the C.A.R.E. program I'm teaching you in this book.

This is particularly true of the methylenetetrahydrofolate reductase (MTHFR) enzyme. The role of this enzyme is to turn folic acid into 5-methyltetrahydrofolate (5-MTHF), otherwise known as folate. Often, in research and in blood test results, folic acid and folate are used interchangeably, so I want to warn you that they are not the same. Folic acid is the inactive form of the nutrient, often used in supplements and fortified foods because it is cheaper. 5-MTHF is the activate form of the nutrient. Approximately 40 percent (or more) of people have at least one of the most researched *MTHFR* gene variations, C677T and A1298C, potentially making them 30 to 80 percent less likely to be able to turn folic acid into folate.

I say "potentially" because when it comes to gene expression, we must always take into account epigenetics, which means stress exposure. To know whether a gene variant is affecting your health, you need to do tests of the actual levels of the metabolites in your body. In the case of MTHFR, we need to measure homocysteine in the blood to know whether there is a lack of methylated folate (5-MTHF). It gets complicated quickly, however, because homocysteine is influenced by many things, including the level of associated nutrients, like B12, as well as stress exposure. Please keep in mind that most practitioners are not trained in this area and standards of care do not yet exist. When I work with patients, I guide them through my protocol step-by-step, individualizing based on their genetics, nutrient levels, and stress exposure.

These gene variations (especially C677T) have been associated with many health issues, including increased risk of miscarriage, migraines, blood clots, anxiety, depression, abnormal pap smear results, and fatigue. Why is this? It's because folate is essential for combining with vitamin B12 (specifically methylcobalamin) in a metabolic process called methylation. I find it helps to think of methylation as a circular process that spins like a wheel based on nutrients coming in and stresses slowing it down. Methylation involves all the B vitamins, which means they are all important, but without active folate, the wheel doesn't turn or turns more slowly; this decreases the production of SAM, which has many important roles in the body, including the protection of DNA from damage by oxidative stress, the production of new healthy cells, detoxification in the liver, and the production and breakdown of serotonin, dopamine, and adrenaline.

If you have one or two variations of the *MTHFR* gene, the best way to detour around the roadblock is to take folate (5-MTHF) instead of folic acid. Check your multivitamin, B complex, or prenatal vitamin to be sure it doesn't contain folic acid. And if it does, replace it. Then have your doctor check the homocysteine level in your blood to determine how well your methylation cycle is working. If it is higher than about 8, this is an indication that stress of some sort is slowing down the process. Once you've addressed the stress, if your homocysteine level is still high, then you can up your dose of 5-MTHF, but I encourage you to go slowly so as not to overwhelm your system. You'll also want to take 5-MTHF with the other necessary B vitamins, including methylcobalamin (B12), riboflavin (B2), and pyridoxine (B6). If your homocysteine level is less than 4, your system is actually depleted and needs recovery from stress before adding more 5-MTHF.

The processing of B vitamins, called methylation, ties into so many other processes in the body, including the metabolizing of adrenaline—that's why B vitamins are so important, especially when we are stressed. And you'll recall that whether our genes are expressing or not is determined by our stress exposure. The more stress we are exposed to, the more likely our bodies are to send more adrenaline down the pathway; at the same time, the more stress we are exposed to, the more likely we are to turn *on* gene variations that cause us *not* to process (get rid of) adrenaline efficiently, which leads to even higher adrenaline levels. So the spiral of stress ensues. Those with this tendency toward higher adrenaline are "good" at responding under stress and tend to choose careers and activities that are more stressful and stress provoking as a result; after all, this is what feels "normal" to them. At the same time, they are more likely to experience adrenal distress.

## A Snapshot of Stress and Illness

It's tempting to blow off the effects of stress. Patients often ask me whether their stress is such a big deal. After all, we all have stress in our lives. True. But that doesn't mean our bodies are able to handle it.

A second problem with this line of thinking is that it implies that those whose bodies become sick from stress are less capable or inferior at dealing with life. This perpetuates patterns of bullying and negative self-talk. And, you guessed it, that creates more stress.

We must be careful about misunderstanding the ramifications of stress. First off, there's a stigma associated with stress and anxiety. You are not "hysterical," nor are you "lazy"—the anxiety and fatigue that you're experiencing are actually symptoms of adrenal distress. Rather than judge others or ourselves for having physical and emotional responses to stress, what if we were to see them as signs that the person is being negatively affected by stress and in need of help to recover? In fact, shifting our view of stress to one of acceptance could break the cycle of stress and decrease both minor and major health issues.

Unfortunately, it's common for people to lump all the symptoms of adrenal distress together and feel overwhelmed by them, as well as by the tendency of practitioners to fail to diagnose patients properly. Patients find themselves going to doctors' offices, seeing specialists, and paying regular visits to the emergency room to find out what's going on—all to no avail. They may be in pain, worried for their health and future, and unable to carry out their daily activities—yet their tests and imaging are all declared "normal." And in many cases, people are given a diagnosis that leads to the prescription of pain medications, antibiotics, steroids, and/or benzodiazepines in an attempt to turn off the symptoms, when in fact it's their adrenal distress that needs to be addressed.

Fibromyalgia, chronic fatigue syndrome, irritable bowel syndrome (IBS), insomnia, and generalized anxiety are all diagnoses often given to people experiencing adrenal distress, and doctors often label patients with these illnesses when there isn't a specific injury or condition to address. When it comes down to it, these conditions are often caused by various types of stress. Medications can be used to mitigate some of the symptoms, but, unfortunately, they won't help people recover from these conditions. They simply mask the symptoms for the time being, and those who take them risk becoming dependent on pills to keep their symptoms from becoming overbearing.

More than one in eight people are addicted to pain medications and/or benzodiazepines, not to mention other substances like sugar and alcohol that we use to get a grip on our stressful reality.[6] Is reaching for a magic pill or comfort food really helping us solve the stress epidemic? Or is it creating more stress that spirals thousands of people each year into eating disorders, substance abuse, and addiction to medications?

In some cases, practitioners actually do tell patients that their condition is due to stress. My mother, who recently had a stroke, was told that her stroke was caused by stress associated with moving from one home to another home, which required months of sorting, packing, cleaning, and unpacking. Yet even when practitioners acknowledge stress as the underlying cause of an illness, they often then leave patients alone with the weight of that information, wondering whether there's anything they can do to prevent future worries.

There's no simple way to eliminate all stress. In fact, we wouldn't want to because stress is an essential part of life. We can make choices to dial it down a bit, and I'll be guiding you on strategic ways to do that through the rest of the book. But we also need to learn how to support our bodies when we are under stress, to recover. What I've found—and this is especially true for people who are willing to make diet and lifestyle changes and want to solve their health issues in order to feel better, improve their quality of life, and potentially extend the length of their lives—is that it is not just about *managing* stress but about *mastering* stress.

## Staying in the Flow

When we begin to experience a health issue, we tend to focus on getting that health issue to go away—the allergic sneezing, the rash on our skin, the headache, the joint pain, the anxiety, or the infection. We look for quick fixes and medications to squash the discomfort as soon as possible.

However, if your stress exposure, cortisol, and adrenaline levels remain the same, the issue will recur. Or more health issues will develop. As long as your body stays in adrenal distress, anything you do is just a temporary fix. Ultimately, you'll be facing dire consequences.

If you really want your health issues to go away, once and for all, you need to identify and address what's causing them in the first place: adrenal distress. Stress without enough stress recovery leaves you susceptible. It disrupts the healthy functions in your body, causing the symptoms and health issues that you are experiencing. It is only when you address adrenal distress and really reset your stress response system that you can truly eliminate your nagging health issues and prevent them from coming back.

The best part: instead of being frustrated and focused on eliminating symptoms, you will start realizing that the symptoms are actually a symbol or an indicator of your stress and the imbalance in your stress hormones. You may even begin to appreciate the symptoms that show up as reminders that you need to get your stress recovery back on track. And once you do get back in balance, then you can focus on keeping yourself that way, which I refer to as stress resiliency.

Let's now turn to the topics of how to determine who is most at risk for adrenal distress, common sources of stress, and why adrenal distress is so often missed and easily dismissed by conventional medicine. We'll also explore the long-term medical, emotional, and even spiritual ramifications of not correcting this state.

3

# What's Stressing You Out?

So, who's most at risk for adrenal distress, and why is this condition so often dismissed by conventional medicine?

The truth is that any person, at any time, and at any age, can be subject to adrenal distress. Stress, and adrenal distress, doesn't discriminate. Remember, in conventional medicine, doctors look for diagnosable conditions that they can treat, which sometimes means prescribing pharmaceuticals—and adrenal distress does not fit that bill. It won't show up on a regular blood test, even though it will affect your long-term health.

## Could You Have Adrenal Distress?

To figure out whether you're at risk, you must consider the *types* of stress you might be under. Understanding stress isn't easy. In fact, one of the most difficult concepts about stress, and your relationship with it, is that there's no "yes or no," "black or white," "one-size-fits-all" way to address it for everyone. It's about finding a balance of what *your* body needs, because everyone's response to stress is different. And this is a hard concept to grasp. As humans, our nature is to turn things all the way off or all the way on, but managing your specific stress levels ultimately means embracing the middle ground.

The most common misconception about stress is that it is brought on only by sudden changes or disruptions in our lives. Yes, the psycho-emotional stress that follows experiences such as death, divorce, and job loss is real. But that isn't the only form of stress in our lives. Stress also follows years of childhood abuse or trauma. Stress is associated with racial and other forms of discrimination. It can infiltrate our lives on a day-to-day basis through the foods that we eat, our sleep patterns, and exposure to toxins in the products we use and the air that we breathe.

At the same time, some experienced stress is necessary. For example, being in labor and having a baby are considered stressful. Yet they're obviously required for human life to continue. Being a parent, especially while juggling a job, can be very stressful, and yet this is a stress that many of us choose to have in our lives. While we often hear about the need for work-life balance, studies suggest that forcing parents to set arbitrary boundaries between parenting and work is actually more detrimental; meanwhile, flexible work arrangements reduce the risk of burnout.[1] Learning how to be okay with stressful, competing needs for our attention is good for our brains and our bodies—and helps prevent adrenal distress.

## Stress from the Past

We tend to think of stress and burnout as psychological issues, but a demanding job and a mile-long to-do list are not the only culprits. Childhood stress can also play a large role in determining whether we develop adrenal distress.

Consider a fascinating piece of research called the Adverse Childhood Experiences (ACE) Study. A survey of over 13,000 adults showed that the more exposure you have to stressful experiences during childhood, the more likely they are to affect your long-term health. In the study, three types of childhood stress exposure were assessed to assign a score: abuse, neglect, and household dysfunction. The higher your ACE score, the higher your risk of diabetes, obesity, depression, suicide attempts, heart disease, cancer, and substance abuse, as well as sexually transmitted diseases and broken bones.[2] Subsequent studies have identified additional childhood experiences that increase health risks and indicate that more than two-thirds of children experience at least one traumatic event before the age of sixteen.[3]

Acknowledging your childhood trauma can be very validating. This doesn't erase the past or necessarily make it any easier to get through life, but it can help you understand your body at this point in time and what you need to do to support your future health. If you know, for example, that your parent abused a substance like alcohol and your parents were divorced, or you were abused, then you can be proactive at this point in your life and prevent that stress exposure from your childhood from negatively affecting your health today.

Again, stress recovery is possible. While the path of your life may not have started off with the optimal amount of nurturing and parental support, this doesn't mean that your health destiny is set in stone—not from what the studies say, and not from what I've seen with my patients.[4] Our bodies and brains are malleable and adaptive. Even when you're exposed to stress, you can give your body the support it needs to recover, getting your cortisol and adrenaline levels back to within normal ranges for feeling good and preventing illness. So don't give up if you had a rough childhood. Don't give up if you feel helpless and caught in a loop of what seems like unending stress triggers. There's a lot that you can do to help your body recover from stress. And if you, like me, are a parent, please know that there's a lot that you can do to help your children recover from their childhood, too. My hope is for this book to help decrease the percentage of children exposed to adverse experiences in future generations by improving our understanding of stress and how to recover from it.

## What We Carry: A Closer Look at Childhood

Compared to children who experience abuse or a major crisis, my daughter has been exposed to a relatively low amount of stress in her childhood. Her father and I were divorced when she was young, which is considered a major stress, yet she has still been able to spend time with both of us, and we have attempted to provide her with an abundance of support, whenever it's needed. Most people would consider this to be a common level of childhood stress in this day and age. Still, my awareness of and research into chronic stress exposure has caused me to rethink how I parent and how I can support my daughter through her stress exposure.

Authoritarian parenting is about obedience, for children to "not speak unless spoken to" and for parents to create rules for children to follow. When the child breaks those rules, the parents enforce consequences, without necessarily having a conversation with the child about why they made the choice they made and how to choose differently in the future. Seldom is there loving or compassionate support, especially during teenage years. Eventually, the teen distances themselves emotionally and physically from the parents and leaves home to create their own life. That said, this type of parenting has been shown to increase the tendency toward anxiety, depression, and digestive health issues—in other words, health issues associated with stress.[5] Furthermore, in most cases under this model, there isn't much chance to discuss or reconcile miscommunications from childhood. If the child does bring up traumatic experiences, it's common for the parents to feel defensive and unappreciated after all they invested in their child.

Thankfully, we have the power to react and respond differently today and to help curtail our children's stress. It's powerful for kids to be seen and heard, and this can influence both the health of the child and the parent. Instead of leaving your child to navigate hardships on their own, take every chance you can to check in with your kids to help them know that all of us have experienced events in childhood that have made us feel invalidated or abandoned. Reinforce that recovery is possible and support is a normal human need that parents can help their children receive. In doing so, you'll change the trajectory of your health, your child's health, and the health of future generations.

In patient reports, I've noticed that adults with low ACE ratings still experience times when they question whether they are "enough" or "lovable" and wonder if certain circumstances were "their fault." I would venture to say that the experience of questioning our own value may be part of human development as we grow toward independence.

Those of us who were exposed to more extreme levels of stress and have higher ACE scores are even more likely to question our own worth. And we're less likely to receive the support and nurturing we need to counteract our past and to develop coping techniques for when our emotional stress is high.

Ultimately, I believe that learning methods to help cope with stress ought to be part of elementary school education. It's that essential for human health. Most parents aren't familiar with these techniques for themselves, let alone their children. To truly shift the negative effect stress is having on our lives, we need to plan ahead and help both adults and children become masters at understanding and supporting themselves so that they can recover from stress of all types.

What's more, studies show that our stress timeline can begin before we are even born! Our bodies and genes reflect stress that we were exposed to in utero and—get this—even stress that our parents and grandparents were exposed to in *their* lives.[6] That means the stress that my grandmother experienced when my grandfather went off to fight in World War II is in my genes. And the stress that my father experienced when his father came back from the war is also in my cells. The toxins that my mother was exposed to on the farm where she grew up influence my body to this day. While this information shocks and amazes me, it is also a powerful call to action.

Studies indicate that just as stressful events, as well as diet and environmental factors, cause epigenetic changes that are inherited in the next generations, positive changes that can assist with stress recovery can be passed on as well.[7] This is of particular interest for men and women who are planning to conceive. More than ever, both sexes have good reason to improve their health before getting pregnant so as to deliver the best genetic expression and highest potential for health to their children.

Many stresses, like those we "inherit," are beyond our control, so we need to be aware of our baselines and work to reduce stress toward them. Studies show that meditation can help.[8] So can prayer. Community support is also a plus. What if we choose to hold each other up in stressful times? What if we prioritize stress recovery (taking a nap, doing a few minutes of yoga, taking a midday walk) instead of viewing it as an indulgence? We must choose nurturance over separation, connection and compassion over discrimination.

## Today's Toxic Stress

We encounter numerous stresses every day that turn our genes on and off. We can, and should, be aware of them, limit exposure, and heal their damage to mitigate their effects on our adrenals.

For starters, toxins in the environment, whether on a farm, in the city, or in the suburbs, are a stress on our bodies. They demand that the liver detoxify them effectively in order to protect our cells and DNA from potential damage. The liver is also responsible for detoxifying estrogens and toxins made by gut bacteria, in addition to medications and alcohol.

Liver detoxification involves CYP450 enzymes, which are influenced by genetic variations and begin turning toxins and chemicals into substances that we can eventually excrete in our feces. For that to happen, the toxic metabolites must first pass through the second phase of liver detoxification, which involves biochemical pathways that further modify the toxins using antioxidants and nutrients, such as B vitamins. These pathways, including methylation and glutathione production, are also greatly influenced by both genetics and stress exposure.

When these pathways are working well, the toxin metabolites are able to exit the liver in bile and pass through the gallbladder and into the intestines, where fiber helps them become part of feces. If the pathways are blocked or not working well, unprocessed toxins can remain in our bodies, increase oxidative stress, and cause damage to our DNA and cells. This increases risk of cancers, neurological damage, dementia, and autoimmunity. Essentially, the more stress and toxins we are exposed to, the less effectively we can detoxify pollutants that enter our bodies.

Many people don't believe that toxins have any kind of negative effect on our health—perhaps because they are invisible. Others simply assume our bodies can handle them. But if we can trace a direct effect from toxins, we're more likely to open our eyes to their larger effects.

For example, if you learned that your mattress was filled with flame retardants and causing vomiting, would that convince you that toxins were having an influence on your health? Or take, for example, what happened to one of my patients, who learned that water had been dripping into her wedding dress box in a closet for a long period of time. Mold grew in the water-damaged box and spewed mold toxins into her home, making her sick. Or consider another patient who accidentally put a drugstore heat pack through her dryer, which caused her to develop debilitating neurological symptoms and forced her to move out of her home and change jobs. Or what about my patients who were present at ground zero on 9/11, an established stressful event and toxic site, and are at increased risk of developing health issues, including dementia and cancer?

The thing is, toxins are everywhere.

They can be in our food in the form of pesticides, additives, colors, preservatives, and flavor enhancers, such as monosodium glutamate (MSG), which acts as a toxin in our nervous system and leads to excessive stimulation by the neurotransmitter glutamate.

Toxins—namely, metals, chlorine, and pharmaceuticals—are present in our water, unless we filter it with a reverse osmosis filter. Irritants and cancer-causing substances from car exhaust, industrial pollutants, and dry cleaning are found in our air, and toxins used in insecticides, building materials, carpets, and furniture are found in our homes (a new home could actually be more toxic than an old one).

Personal care products like lotion, soaps, shampoo, detergents, and perfumes, as well as hair color and nail polish, all potentially contain parabens and phthalates, which are known carcinogens and endocrine disruptors that confuse hormone signaling in our bodies and can predispose us to conditions like endometriosis and fertility issues. Plastics, like those in water bottles, food containers, and toys, can also disrupt hormones in our bodies and act as a stress.

It's not just alcohol, medications, and metals (like mercury in tuna and amalgam dental fillings) that need to be metabolized by our livers. As you can see, we are surrounded by toxins that can overwhelm our detoxification pathways.

## Stress in the Gut

Another major source of toxicity is your very own gut. That's right: your intestines may be adding toxins to your list of insults, due to toxic bacteria

## IN DEPTH: OXIDATIVE STRESS

Oxidative stress is caused by an imbalance between reactive oxygen species (ROS or free radicals) and antioxidants in our body and cells. Redox (reduction-oxidation) reactions, whereby an electron is transferred between two substances, are constantly occurring within our bodies. When these reactions are disrupted by various stresses on our bodies or by toxin exposure, the free radicals are able to cause damage to our cells and DNA, which is what we refer to as oxidative stress. It is essentially stress inside our cells. Our bodies also make antioxidants to counteract oxidative stress, such as glutathione. Some amount of oxidative stress is normal and is necessary; for example, when an infection occurs, ROS are released to signal a protective response from the immune system, known as the inflammasome—creating inflammation to fend off the infection.[9]

The ROS are produced by mitochondria, which are the energy-producing organelles inside our cells. When our mitochondria are triggered by stresses, whether from outside our bodies (such as toxins) or from inside our bodies, they activate mitochondrial hormesis or mitohormesis—a sort of stress defense—which increases mitochondrial performance or functioning, increases antioxidants, and increases detoxification.[10] All of this together prevents damage to our DNA and cells, delays what we think of as "aging," and increases longevity. If, however, the mitochondria are overwhelmed by stress and oxidative stress, mitohormesis decreases, which can lead to negative effects and increase the risk of disease processes such as diabetes and neurodegeneration.[11]

All of this means that the more stressed we are, the more likely we are to have difficulty managing toxin exposure, and the more toxins we are exposed to, the less able we are to handle more stress and toxins. It is a paradox—we might hope that our bodies would have an unending ability to protect us from stress. I find that this vicious cycle of worsening ability to withstand stress follows the mathematical principle of chaos theory. According to chaos theory, otherwise known as the butterfly effect, a small change in a system can result in larger differences later on, due to interconnectedness and feedback loops observed in nature. This is why once health issues begin to develop, the tendency is for more health issues to layer on top of the original issue. Our focus, therefore, must be on giving our bodies the support they need before this process ensues, or on reversing the downward spiral.

overgrowth. Your microbiome includes trillions of bacteria living in your intestines—so much for "being sterile" and thinking you are the only one living in your body! In fact, studies have now identified bacteria that live in all areas of our bodies, including the ovaries, uterus, and bladder.[12] And the bacteria living in us and on our skin contribute more cells to our being than the cells of our bodies. They communicate with our immune and nervous systems to such an extent that they can actually cause us to crave the foods that feed them![13]

The bacteria living in your intestines are affected by stress on your body, which actually began before you were born. And they're further influenced by what you feed them—that is, by what you eat.[14] Eating vegetables, fruit, nuts, and seeds tends to grow bacteria that are best for your health. When you overconsume sugar, grains (wheat, rye, barley, corn, rice), and processed foods, you overfeed bacteria that produce toxins. These substances, called lipopoly-saccharides (LPS), can damage and travel across the intestinal lining, moving into your bloodstream and liver. They can gum up the systems you count on for handling toxins and prevent the effective use of B vitamins for making healthy cells in your body.

Imbalanced gut bacteria, also called dysbiosis, has been associated with almost every health issue in the body, including diabetes; cancer; infections; infertility; menstrual issues like polycystic ovary syndrome (PCOS) and endometriosis; anxiety and depression; weight gain; obesity; skin issues like eczema; and autoimmune conditions like Crohn's disease, rheumatoid arthritis, lupus, and multiple sclerosis (MS). Even osteoporosis, kidney disease, heart disease, and dementia have been linked to an overgrowth of the wrong bacteria in the intestines, and in some cases, the overgrowth of yeast or candida.[15]

It's important to note that it's not harmful when these potentially toxic bacteria and yeasts are present in small amounts. That's why I believe the problem is so often missed in our medical community. Plus, we aren't yet standardly testing for a healthy microbiome in medical care, so most people have no idea what's up with the population of bacteria in their gut. Only naturopathic or functional medicine practitioners run panels to measure the bacteria in patients' intestines based on the bacteria's DNA. Doing a stool test at the regular doctor's office is not going to yield this type of information.

Consider, too, that most pharmaceutical medications, including antibiotics, negatively affect bacterial balance, as do pesticides on foods. Stress can also affect your gut on its own. Studies show that simply being stressed decreases the number of gut bacteria we count on to protect us from our environment; this means that we have fewer bacteria to produce nutrients that we can't otherwise get from our diet, to detoxify toxins in our intestines, to produce neurotransmitters such as serotonin and GABA, and to convert our thyroid hormone to the active form. It's easy to see that stress is a losing game for the gut unless we stay ahead of it and eat in ways that keep the good guys healthy and the bad guys from overgrowing.[16]

All these stresses we're talking about also directly damage the intestinal cells lining the gut walls, which causes what's called intestinal permeability or leaky gut. Once they're leaky, intestinal walls allow undigested food and bacterial toxins to pass through them and into our bodies, where usually only fully digested food, nutrients, and water are allowed to go. Undigested food particles can trigger an immune response, especially given that 80 percent of our immune system is located in our intestines, which then causes a cascade of inflammatory signals throughout the body. Meanwhile, with leaky gut, we absorb fewer nutrients and become susceptible to nutrient deficiency. It makes sense, then, that leaky gut is associated with many conditions tied to inflammation and nutrient deficiencies, such as autoimmunity, allergies, headaches, skin rashes, depression, anxiety, weight gain, joint pain, and brain fog.[17]

Combining dysbiosis with a leaky guy creates the perfect storm of internal stress, which communicates back to the nervous system and triggers even more of a stress response, worsening the issue. Researchers refer to this interplay as the gut-brain axis or gut-brain-microbiome axis because it shows the interconnection between stress, gut health, and health issues throughout the body.[18] Complex health problems become more likely because of the gut-brain axis. When we reverse it, however, by breaking the patterns that are creating the health issues, we can actually use the gut-brain axis to our advantage to speed up healing.

## The Preventive Power of Intentional Eating

Managing your gut might feel like a lot to wrangle on top of an overly busy life. When you're slammed, you're much more likely to eat a high-sugar, high-carb meal in the morning (think of the usual American breakfast of cereal, pancakes, or a donut), add a sugary beverage (juice or a coffee drink), and then rush through the day without much chance to eat again, leading to an oversize dinner. This way of eating is exactly what the LPS-producing bacteria love, and it leads to insulin and leptin resistance, weight gain, and inflammation.

Resistance occurs when a substance, in this case a hormone, no longer triggers its intended response. Insulin is the hormone made by the pancreas that acts like a key to the doorway of our cells, allowing glucose, or blood sugar, to be used as energy. When the amount of glucose in the blood is too high, too often, the cells no longer respond to insulin, referred to as metabolic syndrome, leaving a high amount of glucose in the blood. When the blood circulates through the liver, the excess glucose is turned into fat, which is then put into storage in three possible locations. First, the glucose can be stored in the liver (which can cause a condition known as fatty liver). Second, the glucose can be turned into cholesterol or triglycerides, raising the level of those substances in the blood. Third, the glucose can go into fat storage in the body, often around the waist. Once the liver converts glucose to fat, it is difficult to reverse. Much to our chagrin, the body is more likely to break down muscle for energy than it is to use fat in storage.[19]

Leptin, on the other hand, is the hormone released from fat cells that manages hunger and fullness. It tells our brain when we need to eat and when we've had enough. Eating at odd intervals of time, and in super quantities, throws off leptin signaling. We actually lose track of our hunger and fullness. With leptin resistance, it can seem that we are hungry right after we eat. And it can feel like we are never satisfied, even after an amazing meal. Leptin also signals to the hypothalamus and HPA (stress response) axis. When leptin levels are high (as with leptin resistance), cortisol levels can go even higher and worsen the cycle of stress.

We would like to think that our bodies can self-regulate and use the food we swallow over a long period of time. Our bodies *do* have ways of dealing with whatever we put into them, but those options are not always optimal for our long-term health. Ultimately, it is up to us to choose differently and eat in a way that matches what our bodies need to maintain balance. Instead of allowing yourself to fill your plate with food, or allowing the amount of food you're served to determine how much and when you eat, it's time to start swallowing only what your body can digest, absorb, and use at that time.

When we analyze the ritual of meals through history among various cultures, we see that what was eaten and when it was eaten matches up with what modern science recommends. We need to pair small, predictable quantities of food containing a balance of protein, carbohydrates, and fats with an interval of not eating, usually overnight.

Our busy lives can throw this ideal eating pattern completely to the curb. When this happens, it directly affects our health in a negative way. That's why I consider irregular eating patterns to be a stress. To make matters worse, our bodies don't have a fast way of telling us that we ate enough. The fullness signal can take twenty to thirty minutes to reach our consciousness, and in this time we can eat more food and become overly full. Our bodies also don't have a way to tell us whether we ate enough protein versus fats versus carbohydrates (the three components of food and the three energy sources we depend on to keep us moving, thinking, breathing, and enjoying life). Therefore, it's our responsibility to track these dietary needs so that our bodies can thrive or develop intuitive eating habits.

Finally, trendy eating patterns and extreme diets can throw off our hormones and gut bacteria, triggering a stress response. Many people become so focused on losing weight quickly, and attempting to correct what has gotten out of control, that they swing the other way. They find themselves severely restricting calories and/or fasting for long periods of time, then overeating large meals once the restriction time is done. There are also times when we end up overconsuming foods that are "healthy," such as kale, green juices, avocados, nuts, and/or fermented foods. With such approaches, we can overburden or overstress our guts—more isn't always better. Our bodies need balance.

While there's research behind intermittent fasting (fasting overnight), fasting mimicking diet, and a ketogenic diet, especially for particular health concerns, it's also important to prepare your body first and to monitor and adjust your eating based on how your body responds; otherwise, what is meant to be health producing can become stressful. We'll talk more in future chapters about how to eat, and how to integrate well-researched methods of fasting, in a way that doesn't stress your body even more.

## Too Little Sleep Equals Stress

Have you ever heard someone say, "I'll sleep when I'm dead"? Talk about a lie that conditions us to suffer.

Humans need sleep.

Yet the stresses and demands of life can leave sleep at the bottom of your to-do list—somewhere after you make money to pay your bills and feed your family, clean the house and do the laundry, help your kids with their homework, take care of your pets, call and care for your parents, answer emails and texts, listen to the news, and make sure to wake up in time to catch a flight or get to work the next day.

Even once your head hits the pillow, sleep can be disrupted by lights, noises, children, animals, anxieties, and the need to go to the bathroom. Even if you are able to navigate all of these potential interruptions, your day's stresses and blue-light exposure from your phone and computer decrease melatonin, the sleep hormone produced by the pineal gland. Without adequate melatonin, and with disruptive stress hormones running rampant, it can be really hard to get a good night's sleep even if you adequately prioritize it.

The next thing you know, you might find yourself in the disappointing spiral of insomnia—you know, where you lie down in bed, only to find your mind racing and counting the hours before you have to be up again. At that point, you may find yourself having to choose between being angry at your body for not going to sleep and questioning your whole life and existence. That's when it becomes most apparent why sleep deprivation is a form of torture.[20]

While I loved the training to become a midwife, it also meant I was up all night, several nights each week, for several years. Labor tends to begin right about the time we go to bed! And I was training to be a home-birth midwife, so inevitably my beeper would go off just as I put on my pajamas. I was the first to arrive to assess and support the woman in labor, so there was no time to sleep. When I arrived home after the birth, I couldn't go to sleep because I was getting my doctorate in naturopathic medicine at the same time, so I had classes to attend and patients to see in the clinic. One day, I got in my car and couldn't figure out why it wouldn't start, and then realized, I didn't put the keys in the ignition! That's when I knew, the sleep deprivation had caught up with me and I was showing signs of brain fog and adrenal distress.

Getting less than seven and a half hours of sleep per night is both caused by adrenal distress and a cause of adrenal distress. For those who are able to sleep, the challenge is getting yourself into bed in time for you to be able to get enough sleep before your alarm goes off. And for those who wish they could sleep but are fighting their circadian rhythm, it's a matter of retraining and rebalancing the body systems so that they are signaling sleep at the right time of day.

The good news: these stresses can be avoided or addressed once you know what to pay attention to and match your daily routine and sleep schedule to a less stressful pattern. It is possible to recover (I'm proof!) and I'll show you how. Later in the book, when we turn our focus to practical changes we can make, we'll do just that.

## Stresses Beyond Your Control

In some cases, and at some points in our lives, stress brings us to the point of reconsidering the schedules we've created for ourselves, the jobs we have chosen, and the boundaries, or lack thereof, that we have established for ourselves.

I want to be clear with you that when I share stories about my life, it is not just to talk about me. It is to share with you that I understand the emotional and/or physical pain you are experiencing. I may not have experienced exactly what you've been through, but I do understand what we tend to put ourselves through as humans. Not just what others do to us, but what we end up doing to ourselves because we think we have to or in the name of helping others. I know it can feel very dark and alone. I also know that it cannot be removed with surgery.

While I was writing this book, I had surgery to remove a benign (non-cancerous) growth on my neck. While many doctors told me the surgery was "cosmetic," and even though I tried everything I could think of to avoid having surgery, in the end, the size of the growth and the need to diagnose it led to me having it removed, or at least the part they could reach easily. Meanwhile, through much soul-searching and the tools I'm about to tell you about in this book, I came to the realization that the growth is a consolidation of stress in my body. It is what my body chose to do with the stress it has endured. Surgery removed the lump. Now it is my role, my choice, my life decision to help my body recover. I believe it is possible to follow our life purpose without wearing ourselves out. I want you to know that I am here to be on that journey with you if you choose that for yourself.

There are certainly stressful circumstances that we can't do anything about or that are currently beyond our control. Think financial needs, parenting challenges, relationship struggles, natural disasters, or the death or injury of a loved one.

Consider 2020's worldwide experience of quarantine. It caused us to rethink how we spend our time, how we do our jobs, and even why we leave our homes. Our schedules were completely turned upside down. We were forced into a time of reflection and reevaluation, coupled with the deep distress of a pandemic. Those who traveled or commuted for their jobs were able to find out whether travel was really necessary. Those in the service industry had to think about how to offer those services in a different way. Many people lost their jobs and were in the position of rethinking everything.

Life changed in a snap. And that, in itself, is a stress. The unknown is always a stress. That's why the psychological models of stress always talk about food, water, sleep, shelter, and love as essential needs. If they're not met, we are most certainly stressed. We have to find ways to support ourselves through the stressful situations we can't control. Once we can rise above the stress, or even surf the continual waves of stress, we can see that changes are an opportunity for us to choose differently. After years of commuting to my offices in Manhattan, Connecticut, and Arizona, during the Covid-19 lockdown, I was forced to stay home. At first, it was scary. I cried and felt alone. Then I realized, *Wow, I feel relieved.* I had more time to do what I wanted: to exercise, to produce a podcast called *How Humans Heal*, and to write this book.

I want you to be able to choose what you want to be doing in your life and feel good doing it. Let's move on to identifying your stress type, so you can learn to give your body the support it needs in parts two and three of the book.

# 4

# Know Your Stress Type

Consider how we think of "combating" or "defending" against stress. I like to compare the art of mastering stress to that of mastering a martial art, such as karate or jujitsu. On the surface, martial arts are viewed as a form of self-defense. On a deeper level, however, those who practice martial arts attain a greater understanding of themselves and their vulnerabilities, develop acceptance and compassion for themselves and others, and cultivate a sense of responsibility for what they choose in each moment. Their approach is similar to that of those who master stress.

Consider the Taoist concept of wu wei, which means "effortless action" and is considered to be the noblest path one can take.[1] Instead of fighting stress, we can skillfully and graciously accept it as part of life, along with our human need for food, sleep, exercise, and stress recovery. Instead of thinking of stress management as one more thing on our to-do list, which adds more stress and overwhelm, we can choose to see this other path of stress mastery.

In this chapter, I'm going to describe the five most common stress types I see in my practice: the Stress Magnet, the Night Owl, Sluggish and Stressed, Blah and Blue, and Tired and Wired. You're not going to find this information in any other book or program because I'm the one who figured out there are different stress types. For each type, I'll quickly unpack its adrenal underpinnings, looking at the science and stress patterns behind the behaviors. After that, I'll help you determine your own stress type with a fun and simple quiz. From here, you'll be able to adjust your diet and activities to best support *your* body, help it recover, and develop resilience to stress.

## What's Your Type?

The effects of stress look different for everyone. It's important to realize that you will respond uniquely to stress and require different support to recover than another person might. As we learned in the last chapters, past stress exposure and genetics play an essential role in determining how stress affects you. They also affect your stress recovery strategies.

After reviewing thousands of cortisol, adrenaline, and neurotransmitter patient results over the past two decades, I started picking up on patterns. Not just patterns among different patients but also repeated patterns in the same patient over time. What I found is that each person has a signature stress pattern, which is essentially how their body responds to stress in terms of whether their cortisol shifts to higher or lower levels earlier or later in the day, and whether their adrenaline goes higher or dips lower. These stress patters correlate with the five stress types.

Remember that each person's stress is determined both by their stress exposure and their genetic tendencies. And each stress type requires a different approach, in terms of diet and lifestyle changes, as well as nutrients and herbs, to help shift cortisol and adrenaline back to optimal levels. By identifying and understanding these stress patterns, we can anticipate, on an individual basis, what is needed to master stress over time.

Let's look now at the five types and their corresponding stress patterns.

## One: The Stress Magnet

### Elevated cortisol with elevated adrenaline in the morning or all day

The Stress Magnet has high adrenaline and high cortisol part or all of the day. They are likely to experience digestion issues, hormone imbalances, and anxiety. These patients feel a constant need to go, all the time, with little rest and recovery.

The Stress Magnet tends to wake up in a state of panic, and often earlier than they'd like to wake up for the day. They describe mind-racing thoughts as soon as they open their eyes, or even before, thinking of everything they need to get done, plus every call and decision they need to make. Some people even find themselves sitting up in bed with a rush of anxiety, or dread, searching for anything to calm themselves down.

If you have this stress pattern, you feel like your mind is pulling you forward while rushing to get you dressed and get your day started. Obviously, you have a million things to get done . . . all before noon. You may feel like you always have another deadline, due date, meeting to plan, project to complete, or conflict to resolve.

Or perhaps you're living in or with a situation that causes unending stress. What began, then, as stress may have caused a health issue that's creating even more stress. Anorexia, insomnia, anxiety, obsessive-compulsive disorder, inflammatory bowel disease (IBD), and cancer (or precancer) are common for this stress type. Health issues themselves can spin a vicious cycle of stress that piles cortisol and adrenaline on top of more cortisol and adrenaline. The next thing you know, you feel like you're running on a never-ending treadmill, racing through each day as if trying to escape from a perpetually angry lion.

People in this stress type tend to choose high-stress jobs. They are willing to do more, push harder, and work longer. They are used to working out and even fasting for long hours. This person may actually feel like they want to continue moving at their customary speed. They are used to the rush or even addicted to this pattern of stress response. They can't imagine life any other way, which makes it harder to implement changes.

But at some point, all this pressure begins to catch up with them. Anxiety increases and weight either decreases or increases, despite skipping meals and exercising. Then they start to feel exhausted. Low moods; digestive issues like constipation or reflux; and viral infections such as flu viruses, human papillomavirus (HPV), or Epstein-Barr virus (EBV) kick in.

In this stress type, high cortisol suppresses healthy digestion and the absorption of nutrients, which leads to nutrient deficiencies along with imbalanced gut bacteria. It also decreases insulin function and increases blood sugar levels, making weight gain and other health issues (fatty liver, decreased memory, and heart disease) more likely. High cortisol also decreases hormone production in the thyroid, ovaries, testes, and more. It also throws off immune function.

My patient Cindy is the perfect example of a Stress Magnet. At fifty years old, she was extremely busy as a school principal, wife, and mother. She was under a tremendous amount of stress at work, particularly during the Covid-19 pandemic. Her day started early, in order to get her young daughter to school and then be at school herself for work. She slept fine when she exercised and took melatonin; otherwise, she'd be up all night. At night, Cindy had heart palpitations, and her history of breast cancer, a hysterectomy, celiac disease, and severe allergies told me that her body had been under stress for a long time. Genetic tendencies to autoimmune conditions like celiac disease, allergies, and cancer turn on when cortisol has been elevated for years.

She saw different practitioners to address her medical issues and make diet changes. Still, none of that got at the real underlying issue: stress. The same cortisol and adrenaline that helped her get through each day also set her up for more and more health issues.

Cindy didn't have to quit her job to heal. (If she had, though, she could have recovered much faster because she could have used the time she spent working to support her health.) Instead, I supported her in counteracting the stress even when she was still stressed. It was critical to give her body clear signals on when it could turn down the cortisol and adrenaline, and use specific approaches on a daily basis to retrain her system to function without being in stress mode. She'll always have the tendency toward being a Stress Magnet, but she's learning how to prevent it from ruining her health.

I find the Stress Magnet type to be common for patients who work in the financial world. Whether it involves making investments and trades all day or working on high-profile mergers, this type of work attracts people who have the ability to maintain high cortisol and adrenaline (based on their genetics and stress history); they then perpetuate the pattern by working long days and taking few days off. One such patient recently came to see me to help her reverse abnormal cells on her cervix, which had showed up on her recent pap smear, due to HPV. Another is an eighty-six-year-old patient who has run his own financial firm for his entire career and still works most days, keeping up with the latest stock market trends. He came to see me for help with severe anxiety, which wasn't helped by the medications he was taking. He also had a history of cancer and digestive issues.

It's important to note that while most people assume they have high cortisol and adrenaline, most don't. And those who do have high cortisol all day long and into the evening, along with high adrenaline, feel awful. They essentially have a combination of Stress Magnet and Night Owl (which you'll read about next) tendencies, setting them up for severe fatigue, the inability to sleep more than an hour or two at a time, off-the-chart anxiety, joint pain, digestive disturbances, and very often anorexia or other eating disorders as well as obsessive-compulsive tendencies.

Quite simply, without a break from stress, all systems start shutting down for Stress Magnets. They start to lose track of what "normal" is because the stress pattern has become their new "normal." I've helped these patients recover, but it becomes more difficult the longer they live in stress mode. That's why I'm so passionate about helping you get out of stress mode before it spirals to this degree.

## Two: The Night Owl

### Elevated cortisol in the evening with elevated adrenaline

In this pattern, a person may feel relatively fine all day, or even perhaps a bit groggy due to staying up late the prior evening. And then, usually after 5 or 6 PM, they'll get a boost in energy. All of a sudden, they feel like getting things done—making dinner, doing laundry, cleaning the house, making calls, and checking things off their to-do list, as well as sitting in front of the computer, surfing or crunching out a project.

Finally, when it is time to go to bed, this person may lie awake, staring at the ceiling or watching YouTube, despite their desire to fall asleep. Their mind and body are literally so alert at bedtime that it's as though they are living in the wrong time zone.

The Night Owl has trouble sleeping because their cortisol and adrenaline levels are highest in the evening. This might happen naturally if you're subject to too much stress during the day, which makes your body unable to "turn off" in the evening. It can also be the result of pushing yourself too late into the night to finish work. All of this can put you into adrenal distress because you're pushing your cortisol too hard, at the wrong time of day.

Here, your days may feel like they last forever, as you drudge your way through the tasks on your list. Until that evening second wind comes in.

Instead of going to bed, you feel like knocking things off the list for tomorrow. Perhaps the kids finally went to sleep, and you have time to focus and think. Or perhaps you've worked two shifts—the day shift and the evening shift—for so many years that your body kicks right back into gear and gets you ready to accomplish a whole other list of to-dos: finish the laundry, reply to emails, shop online, write an article, or watch a TV series and message a friend. Next thing you know, it's 3 AM, and you've got to get up for your next "shift" in a few hours—to drive the kids to school, be at a meeting, get to the airport, or whatever else is on the calendar.

Essentially, you're burning the candle at both ends, whether you like it or not.

This reminds me of my patient Marianne. She's fifty-five years old and a teacher, mom of college-age daughters, and wife. She loves her job as a music and theater teacher, though when it is time to put together a performance, she works around the clock. Marianne's anxiety got so high at one point, in fact, that she had trouble sleeping and developed heart palpitations. Right when she needed to feel her best, stress took over and she felt worse than ever. In a sense, she worked two shifts between her day job and after-school responsibilities. Marianne stayed up late with rehearsals or preparing details of the show and just couldn't turn her mind off because she worried about every detail. When she traveled, she struggled with digestive and menopausal issues, and her body couldn't keep up with all its fluctuations. She went from high cortisol/adrenaline before menopause to low cortisol/adrenaline after menopause. Now both are high at night because she has been working on a theater production and helping her daughters move to their own apartments.

This is characteristic of a Night Owl's stress patterns because the body adapts in a way to help us keep up with superlong days, one after the next. Sometimes our own choices set us up for this pattern, as Marianne's did. We choose a challenge, which is often also our passion, and it requires us to have higher cortisol and adrenaline into the evening.

For others, this can happen without necessarily having a task at hand, or not one that seems apparent. For one patient it happened after changing her career and moving to a new home. All of a sudden, her body went into Night Owl mode. Even though she actually had more time in her life to take care of herself, it was as if her system went into shock after so much change occurred in such a short period of time. Another patient experienced a shift in her body after visiting family due to a relative's death. While she felt she had processed the grief, her body went into Night Owl mode for a couple of months before it settled back to a regular pattern. Yet another patient ran internet security for a major TV station for decades and was on call in the evenings. His body was required to be in Night Owl mode based on his stress exposure and need to work nights. Even once he retired, his body stayed in Night Owl mode—that is, until he met with me and we implemented a recovery plan.

## Three: Sluggish and Stressed

### Elevated cortisol with low adrenaline

Sluggish and Stressed is a variation on the Stress Magnet, but with low adrenaline. Here, patients have a long history of feeling stressed, and it presents as skin rashes, hair loss, digestive issues, anxiety, brain fog, allergies, joint pain, and/or sleep issues.

This person often feels like they've tried everything to feel better and can't seem to hack it. They've experimented with diets, supplements, medications, and exercise strategies, and they still don't feel well or only feel okay for short periods of time.

The Sluggish and Stressed person might wonder if they have attention deficit hyperactivity disorder (ADHD) and might wish that they had more stamina to exercise and get things done. Inflammation is often high, which causes pain, swelling, anxiety, weight gain, decreased memory, low mood, and low inspiration. They are not digesting food well and often feel bloated. While there's so much they would like to do, their body and mind won't allow for it. They often choose sugar and/or caffeine to keep them going throughout the day.

This pattern is more common after decades of stress, whether from work or relationships. This person often feels better when they make a change in their job or relationship, but then they can start to feel worse again if they don't implement supportive strategies. They feel like a slave to their health and body and wish they could enjoy their life.

Patricia, my sixty-seven-year old patient, is a classic Sluggish and Stressed type. She remembered having a lot of energy as a child and when she was younger, but once she hit midlife, her body only wanted to sit still and read. She forced herself to walk for exercise. While the exercise used to energize her, Patricia now felt exhausted by it. By the end of her day, she felt beat from walking up and down her home's stairs and doing daily chores. She struggled with depression and anxiety, low libido, and lack of motivation and was altogether pooped.

Here, Patricia's Sluggish and Stressed pattern was obvious. Because her cortisol was higher in the morning, she often woke up feeling like she was ready to accomplish the tasks on her list and enjoy the day by playing with her grandchildren. But then by midday, even after several cups of coffee to boost her adrenaline, everything came to a halt. What seemed like a great idea suddenly had to be put on the "maybe tomorrow" list.

My patient Daniel is a lawyer who's had his own law practice for almost three decades. He struggled with digestive issues (reflux in particular), allergies, anxiety, and fatigue and sought out and tried all kinds of diet changes and supplements. But nothing seemed to really help him turn the corner. That was, until we identified his problems with leaky gut, imbalanced gut bacteria, and high cortisol in the morning, which perpetuated the gut issues and caused high inflammation both in his joints and in his nervous system (causing anxiety). Even though he had energy to help his clients, he had underlying fatigue due to low adrenaline. Once we solved that, he felt like he had turned back time and was reinspired to succeed in his business and life.

## Four: Blah and Blue

### Low cortisol in the morning or at midday, with low adrenaline

The Blah and Blue type feels tired, depressed or anxious, and unmotivated all day. This person wakes up with low cortisol and/or adrenaline. They immediately feel like pulling the blankets back over their head. In this stress type, adrenal distress is also linked to loneliness and a sense of isolation, which only adds to the stress a person feels.

It's morning? Time to get up? Forget it—you want to hit the snooze button one more time, hoping that eventually you'll get a burst of energy that jolts you out of bed to face the day. It feels like you were hit by a truck or that your body is made of lead. Your limbs feel too heavy to move, and your mind is mush. You may have thoughts like, "What day is it again?" and "How am I going to accomplish even one thing on my to-do list?"

As you make your way to the bathroom, you wish you could head back to bed, or you may even talk yourself into pushing on by thinking that you can take a nap partway through the day. You drink coffee, hoping that it will give you a boost to be somewhat functional, but still your mind feels like it is in mud and your mood is in the tank. You wonder what you can do to possibly feel better when even taking a walk feels impossible.

Alternatively, the low cortisol and adrenaline can occur in the afternoon, after you have put in a full day of work. At this point you feel like you need a nap, but often you need to push to keep going. I tend to see this pattern in patients who have done a lot of commuting and traveling for work, and who are juggling many responsibilities, such as parenting, helping their own parents out, or running a nonprofit organization, alongside their usual activities.

You may feel like your brain gets foggy. You may even feel dizzy or get a migraine right when you have a long list of things to get done; essentially, your body makes it impossible to continue until you get some rest.

My patient Hayley is the epitome of Blah and Blue. At forty years old, she slept twelve hours a night, hit snooze for a half hour each morning (she set five alarms to be sure she got up to make it to work at her job on a TV show as a meteorologist, which she loved), and yawned nonstop during the day. While she often fell asleep on the sofa at 10 PM, she typically made midnight her official bedtime. She described herself as a type A personality, a workaholic who multitasked all day and was willing to take on more. If she wasn't working, then she felt depressed and was prone to mood swings that made her feel anxious or sad.

Hayley's adrenal distress patterns? Low cortisol most of the day and low adrenaline. Low cortisol and adrenaline in the morning made it almost impossible for her to get out of bed. Her genetics and stress exposure set her to feel drained and as if the rug were slipping out from under her. She had low thyroid function and struggled with digestive issues as well, both of which are common when cortisol is low. Like a Stress Magnet, she was drawn to taking on more stress in her body, but instead of shifting to high cortisol and high adrenaline, her body went the opposite way, to low cortisol and low adrenaline.

## Five: Tired and Wired

### Low cortisol morning or midday with elevated adrenaline

Now, this is an interesting mix. The Tired and Wired type has the get-up-and-go from adrenaline combined with the sluggishness of a low-cortisol profile.

If you are the Tired and Wired type, anxiety is your predominant mood, each and every day. It may be so common to feel worried and nervous that it seems normal to you. Making decisions, even about what to have for breakfast or whether to make a phone call, is difficult because your mind is giving you so many things to consider. If you use the eggs now, will you have enough for later? How are you going to find time to get to the grocery store and the bank before you have to be back home? It's like each day is a flood of options, very few of which you can choose before the next day starts the process all over again.

At the same time, you feel too tired to muster the energy to really care or make enough progress for it to matter. With your heart racing, your chest feeling tight, and your mind ruminating, you may actually be good at getting a lot done during the day, but then you find yourself completely spent by 5 PM. You survive by cooking one day a week, stocking up enough food for the other days, and putting everything on repeat so that you don't have to think or decide.

I often find this pattern to be common for working moms, people who are experts in their fields, people who are running businesses, and people who hold jobs with a lot of responsibility. Those with this stress pattern often feel like they're treading water. They may be reluctant to make changes for fear of causing everything to fall apart.

While they can respond under stress to get a task done, underneath it all they are struggling to keep going. Their immune system and hormones often show signs of depletion or overresponsiveness, such as allergic reactions. Yet for these people, it's tempting to look past the initial health issues and try to carry on.

My patient Fatimah is the epitome of the Tired and Wired type. A civil engineer with a high-stress job, two children, and a husband, she had a packed schedule from morning to night. Then she did it all again. At thirty-three years old, she felt drowsy after a night's rest, though she often slept only four or five hours a night because she woke up so early to exercise or meditate. While Fatimah's morning fatigue decreased throughout the day, her anxiety tended to kick in when she had a pressing deadline or didn't feel like she was being productive.

Fatimah's low cortisol levels showed me that her adrenals were struggling to keep up with her highly disciplined routine. To make up for the lack of cortisol, her adrenals overproduced adrenaline, to help keep her going. Her body was adapting to stress and giving her all it had, yet at the same time it was leaving her vulnerable. Human papilloma virus (HPV) kept showing up on her pap smear, and while we were able to turn the abnormal cells around with diet changes and supplements, she knew that it would be back again if she didn't get her body out of prolonged stress mode. Luckily, she made time for important self-care, including exercise, meditation, prayer, and making healthy meals ahead of time for herself and her family. Without these steps in place, she might have succumbed to even more anxiety and health issues.

## Stress types

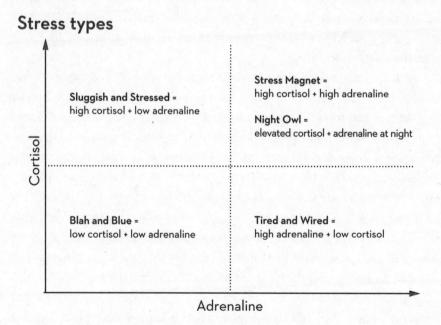

## Feeling a Little Déjà Vu?

Do any of the above patterns feel familiar? None of them are more common at any certain age, and they are not based on sex, race, or where you live in the world. They seem, as far as I can tell from my research and clinical experience, to be the most common responses to stress among *all* humans.

You may be wondering what makes it more likely that you'll land in any one of these patterns or stress types. I've found it seems to be related to a combination of genetic factors, including cortisol and adrenaline production and breakdown, as well as your history of stress exposure.

I see patients of all ages. I've found that children and teens are just as likely to have high or low cortisol and adrenaline as a seventy-five-year-old who's been working in Manhattan's high-stress financial district their whole life. I think this is because children these days are likely to have very full schedules, participating in athletics, performing in plays, excelling in advanced classes, and dreaming of future plans; they are under quite a lot of stress, often self-imposed. As a result, they can experience headaches or migraines; acne; anxiety; sleep issues; nausea; vomiting; inflammatory bowel issues; menstrual irregularities; and autoimmunity, especially after infections like sinus infections, mono, and strep.

At the same time, patients in their sixties, both men and women, often find themselves overwhelmed by a list of developing health issues, including fatigue, low mood, high blood pressure, weight gain, decreased focus, impaired memory, and decreased libido—all combined with less sleep and blood sugar levels that are creeping up. They are often compelled to care for aging parents near or far or to commit years to managing a deceased parent's estate (while also managing siblings), with the fear of aging in the backs of their own minds. What's more, it becomes clear to them that diabetes, cancer, heart attacks, strokes, and dementia are possible outcomes for themselves. After a lifetime of working hard and raising a family, their focus turns inward, and they realize that stress really has done a number on their bodies.

No matter what the scenario, however, we are not alone with these stress patterns. And we can heal. Mastery, though, takes vigilance. In fact, I find that after I help a person recover from stress, getting their cortisol and adrenaline levels back on track, they might find themselves yet again in a highly stressful situation down the road. At this time, their body reverts *right back to the same pattern* they just recovered from. For instance, if they had high cortisol in the morning (and/or at night) and elevated adrenaline, their body will shift right back into that same familiar stress mode. The good news here is that now the stressed-out person knows what to do to recover and get their cortisol and adrenaline back to the levels that allow them to best perform daily tasks and feel good doing it. Having learned their body's stress response pattern, they heal more quickly.

That said, there are rare cases when the body changes to a different stress pattern. Suddenly the Stress Magnet becomes the Blah and Blue. I often see such shifts happen when a person hasn't fully addressed their stress or when a life transition happens, such as menopause. The person may have taken steps to support their adrenals to either make less or more cortisol, but various forms of stress still presided. Perhaps a loved one faced a serious health issue that demanded their time and attention. Or perhaps their job required a move. Maybe they found out that they were getting exposed to mold or another toxin and simply didn't have the time and energy at that moment to help their body recover. In these scenarios, the amount of stress outweighed the anti-stress so much that their stress pattern might have shifted to a more depleted state, like to lower cortisol and/or adrenaline. If they started out with low cortisol and adrenaline, the levels might have gone even lower.

## Self-Assessment

You might be tempted to self-diagnose your stress type immediately, based on the descriptions I provided above. Even so, I encourage you to still take the following self-assessment quiz to confirm your instincts. The results may surprise you, not least of all because chronic stress can change how we view ourselves! Adrenal distress can alter self-awareness, too.

The best way to identify your stress type is by looking at the five areas of your health and well-being most affected by cortisol and adrenaline shifts. These are your energy level and stamina; sleep hours and timing; mental focus and memory; mood; and body symptoms. Remember, cortisol is a hormone that signals to our digestion, immune system, nervous system, and all the other hormones in our bodies. When cortisol shifts, those systems will also be shifted. Adrenaline, on the other hand, is a neurotransmitter, signaling to our bodies to respond to stress. When the levels of cortisol and adrenaline shift, it affects our energy, sleep, focus, mood, and body in general.

As you answer the questions in the quiz, think of how you feel today and have felt over the past week. While you may want to answer these questions based on how you felt when you were under stress or experiencing health issues, I encourage you (at least for your first time through the test) to think of how you feel *right now* and have felt in the past twenty-four to forty-eight hours. We want to essentially take a cross-sectional view of your adrenal distress at this point in time. By knowing where you are now, we can best build a plan for support and recovery.

## Quiz Time!

Below you will find questions separated into five areas: energy, sleep, focus, mood, and body. Each question has five possible answers, numbered one through five. Ask yourself each question in each section, choose the answer that describes you best, and circle that number.

At the end of the quiz, I'll show you how to unpack the results.

### *Energy*

**A. When I think of my energy level in general, I would say:**

1. I have a lot of energy, especially in the morning. My energy can drop midway through the day.
2. My energy level increases in the evening and/or when trying to go to sleep.
3. My energy level varies and is lower than I'd like it to be.
4. It is hard to wake up and get out of bed. I feel exhausted in the morning and/or like I need a nap in the middle of the day.
5. My energy level is okay or low, but I push through.

**B. When I wake up in the morning, my energy level is:**

1. High! I have a lot of energy, especially in the morning.
2. Lower than it will be later in the evening or at night.
3. Unpredictable, but generally lower than I would like it to be.

4. Very low. I feel exhausted and it's hard to get out of bed.
5. Okay or low. I make it through the day on adrenaline.

## C. Throughout the day, my energy level:

1. Makes people think of me as someone who gets a lot done, although my energy can drop a bit midway through the day.
2. Is low, but then it increases in the evening, keeping me awake and getting things done.
3. Is up and down. I often feel I need a nap or caffeine to keep going.
4. Stays low even after a nap and caffeine. It's difficult to exercise.
5. Stays okay or low, but I can exercise and get everything (almost everything) on my to-do list done.

## D. In the evening, my energy level:

1. Is pretty good, actually. I can work a very long day and into the evening.
2. Increases, which can make it hard to fall asleep and stay asleep.
3. Is lower, and I prefer an early bedtime.
4. Is as low as, or lower than, it is the rest of the day. I can't wait to go to bed, even though I know I'll likely wake up tired.
5. Starts to drop, but it's hard for me to calm my mind to go to sleep.

## Sleep

### A. When I think of my sleep in general, I would say:

1. I find that six or seven hours of sleep feels like plenty and I tend to wake up early.
2. I find it difficult to fall asleep, tend to stay up late, or wake up after a couple of hours of sleep.
3. I'm tired in the evening and fall asleep easily, but never feel like I got enough sleep.
4. I can sleep eight hours, but I still wake up tired.
5. I'm tired in the evening and ready for bed, but my mind can race or wake me up.

**B. At 10 PM, I feel like:**

1. I can keep working to finish a project if needed.
2. I wish I could go to sleep, but my body and/or mind are keeping me awake.
3. I wish I could do more, but my body is exhausted.
4. I'm so tired—I'm ready to crash in bed.
5. I'm ready for bed, but it can be difficult to turn my mind off.

## Focus

**A. When I think of my ability to focus, in general, I would say:**

1. I am very energetic, focused, and decisive, and I am able to get lots done, although sometimes I feel overwhelmed.
2. I wake up (even in the middle of the night) with a rush of thoughts or even anxieties. Then it's hard to focus during the day.
3. I have brain fog often and/or need coffee to stay focused.
4. It's very hard to think or get things done. It feels impossible to accomplish the items on my to-do list.
5. I feel overwhelmed by having so much to do. My mind races and I'm easily distracted.

**B. During the middle of the day, my focus:**

1. Is quite good. I can work on several projects at the same time, although I don't always get to finish them all simply because I have so much to do and so little time.
2. Is not good. I feel like a zombie because I don't sleep well. It's hard to focus and my memory has decreased.
3. Is okay, in spurts. Then I get tired and feel like I need a nap.
4. Is a challenge. I wish my brain would work better, but I'm just so tired.
5. Is better than that of others around me, but not perfect. I have to work hard or drink caffeine to keep focused.

## Mood

**A. In regard to my mood, in general, I would say:**

1. I often feel anxious or worried. I can also easily become irritable and annoyed.
2. I feel anxious or irritable at night when trying to sleep.
3. I feel anxious or depressed in the morning or at midday.
4. I wake up with a low mood and low motivation, or anxiety, and it can last all day.
5. I think through what happened, or is about to happen, over and over. I tend to worry.

**B. When I wake in the morning, my mood is:**

1. Often in a state of overwhelm, whether with things to get done or a low mood. I try to push my mood aside in order to get things done.
2. Grumpy, because I didn't sleep well, as usual.
3. All right, but it soon wavers. I feel like I should be able to feel better, which causes me to feel frustrated and alone.
4. Rather low. I prefer to stay by myself, and I do better with a slow start to my day.
5. Good, except that I feel anxious that I won't have time to get everything done.

## Body

**A. When I think of how my body feels, I would say:**

1. I notice my heart racing or feel tightness in my chest during the day.
2. I wake in the night with my heart and mind racing. I get nausea and have trouble gaining (or losing) weight.
3. I tend to gain weight around my waist and have digestive issues.
4. I often feel light-headed or like I might faint. I have cold hands and feet, and I feel worse after exercising.
5. My blood sugar levels drop quickly. I have muscle tightness/tension.

**B. The most common symptoms I feel in my body are:**

1. Heartburn, heart pounding, and mood fluctuations.
2. Weakness and brain fog, from not sleeping well.
3. Joint and/or muscle pain and frequent infections.
4. Fatigue, cold hands and feet, and lack of stamina.
5. Heart racing and recurring infections.

## How to Interpret Your Stress Type

For each section, notice which numbered answer (one to five) most often described you best. Now compare between the five sections. Is there a numbered answer (one to five) that you consistently or more often chose? That number signifies your dominant stress type.

1. Stress Magnet
2. Night Owl
3. Sluggish and Stressed
4. Blah and Blue
5. Tired and Wired

## TESTING YOUR LEVELS

There are clinical panels you can ask your naturopathic doctor or functional medicine practitioner to run for you to assess the function of your adrenal glands. I refer to this type of test as a "stress test" because it shows how your body has been affected by the stress you've been exposed to up to this point in your life. Keep in mind that these panels should be run in addition to the blood tests and imaging a conventional medical practitioner or endocrinologist would order.

Conventional tests for adrenal function show only your fasting blood levels of cortisol in the morning, which is usually useful only for extremely high or low levels—the overproduction or total lack of production of cortisol. Most of us are somewhere in the middle, however,

KNOW YOUR STRESS TYPE

where our adrenals are still making adrenaline and cortisol, but at non-optimal levels at different times of day, so that our bodies feel off in various ways. This likely won't show up on a cortisol blood test, so you may be told that everything is "normal" when clearly you don't feel normal or well.

When, instead, we measure cortisol at four different times of day (upon waking, at midday, in the evening, and at bedtime), we can gather more data to render a more accurate assessment of adrenal distress. I also strongly suggest doing a urine panel to check dopamine, norepinephrine, epinephrine, serotonin, and GABA levels; this way you and your practitioner can see your adrenaline production and neurotransmitter levels. Knowing and addressing your neurotransmitter levels makes stress recovery more effective and efficient.

I prefer to be able to refer to all of these levels in my practice so that I can precisely assess how stress has affected a patient's body. From there I am able to determine their unique response to stress and what is needed to help them recover from it. Cortisol can be reoptimized using specific nutrients and herbs. Adrenaline and neurotransmitters can be rebalanced using nutrients and amino acids, which I'll discuss in part three of this book.

In addition to measuring cortisol, adrenaline, and neurotransmitters, practitioners can run additional tests to help you understand the effects of stress on your body. Because leaky gut and imbalanced gut bacteria are so common with stress exposure, I suggest doing specialty tests to determine how much of an issue they are for you.

The best way to identify leaky gut is with a food sensitivity panel that checks for IgA and IgG antibodies to common foods. This is because our immune system tends to make immune responses to undigested foods that have leaked through the intestinal lining. While there are urine and blood tests to estimate the increase of leakage through the intestinal wall and identify proteins involved in leaky gut, I find that doing a highly accurate food panel provides the information we need about whether leaky gut is present and to what degree, while also showing us exactly which foods are currently triggering inflammation.

IgA and IgG antibodies are delayed-response antibodies, so you're not likely to notice which foods you are reacting to in the moment. This type of antibody response is different from that of IgE antibodies, which trigger immediate allergic responses that you'd find by seeing an allergist. Also, these IgA and IgG tests are not run (or not run well) by regular labs and are rarely covered by insurance. Still, I believe the information we gain from them is essential for stress recovery. You need to know which foods are stressful for your body and therefore which foods to eliminate from your diet while you recover from stress and heal leaky gut. The intention is not to avoid the reactive foods forever. Quite the opposite. The goal is to heal your digestion so that you can go back to eating the foods you enjoy. Gluten is often the only exception, and that is because it is known to cause leaky gut and inflammation, which lead you right back to a stressed state.

As for measuring gut bacteria that could lead to health issues, one of the coolest developments in the past decade has been tests that measure the different types of bacteria in the stool, which reflect the large intestinal microbiome, based on the bacteria's DNA. That means we don't have to rely on a culture, in which bacteria are grown in a lab over a number of days and in multiple stool samples. With a single stool collection, you and your practitioner can find out what is living in your intestines and whether you are digesting your food well, too.

Depending on your stress exposure, you may also need to test for toxins, such as mold toxins, metals, and environmental toxins like those from exhaust fumes, off-gassing, and plastics, all of which can be measured in urine. We can check on metabolites in urine that are related to an effective use of nutrients and mitochondrial function (as discussed earlier, mitochondria are the little energy-producing engines in each one of our cells). We can assess levels of oxidative stress by checking a urine biomarker called 8-hydroxy-2'-deoxyguanosine (8-OHdG), which is released when there is damage to our DNA.[2] We can also measure hormones in the urine, such as estrogen, progesterone, testosterone, dehydroepiandrosterone (DHEA), and melatonin, to find out how hormones have been affected by stress.

In blood, we can check on thyroid function, nutrients, and methylation (how the body uses B vitamins). For thyroid, ask your practitioner to check thyroid-stimulating hormone (TSH), free T3, and free T4, and also to check for thyroid antibodies. To check your iron levels, ask for ferritin, which reflects iron storage. Be sure to ask for homocysteine and methylmalonic acid instead of B12 and folate levels, in order to get an accurate sense of whether you need more B6, B9 (folate), and B12. Vitamin D can also be checked at a regular lab, but for an accurate look at the rest of your nutrients, you'll want to go to a lab that measures intracellular nutrient levels rather than what is floating through the bloodstream.

We can also run genetic panels, using a saliva sample, to identify gene variations that are related to nutrient needs, detoxification, metabolism of neurotransmitters, and more. I particularly like to know whether my patients have variations in the genes *MTHFR, MTRR, COMT, MAO, CYP, VDR, PEMT, CBS*, and *NOS* (to name a few). By knowing my patients' genetic susceptibilities, I can guide them to detour around them using specific nutrients introduced in a certain order. More than anything, it is important to understand that no matter what your gene variations, solving your health is a matter of knowing that various stresses cause your genetic susceptibilities to express, and that stress bogs down your metabolic processes on top of any genetic influence. By simply flipping that around, you can solve health issues. As you recover from and master your stress, you'll be able to lift the slowdowns caused by stress and reset your genetic expression.

There is so much that you can know about your body and how it's been affected by stress that it is mind-blowing. Keep in mind that the tests I've described are not tests that you'll likely find offered by your general practitioner, and most are not covered by insurance, so you'll be forced to think of this form of health care—your stress recovery care—as a separate part of your budget. I suggest you put it in your "self-care" budget, along with the time and money you'll need to spend on stress recovery activities. After all, without your health, what do you have? It's time to take good care of you.

## What Now?

Now that you have identified your stress type, it's time to dig into what can help you get out of stress mode and back to feeling good. Remember that it is possible to shift your cortisol and adrenaline levels back toward optimal registers, for all stress types.

Knowing your stress type is like knowing the "trend" of your body's function; it is similar to knowing a business or financial trend. Once you know the trend, or the tendency to shift toward a certain pattern, you'll be able to anticipate, plan, and choose your daily activities and supplements to help keep your body on point, precisely at the cortisol and adrenaline levels that best serve you and your health.

The good news is that once you know your stress pattern or stress type, I can guide you to recover and not just manage stress but ultimately master it. There are activities, ways of eating, support for sleeping, herbs, nutrients, and other naturally derived substances that help your body and your adrenal function improve and remain in an optimal range. These can allow you to stay healthy, *even while stressed*. Let's dig into part two of the book, where we'll explore individual approaches to helping your body climb out of stress mode through a simple acronym: C.A.R.E.

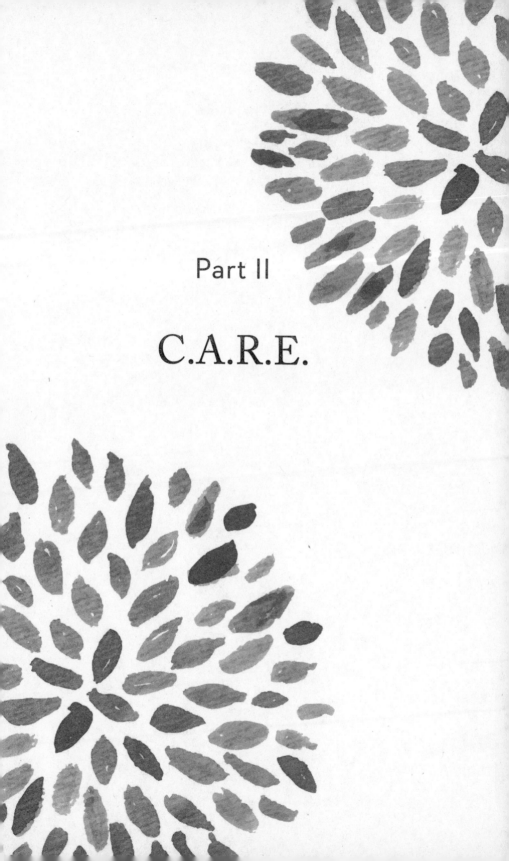

Part II

# C.A.R.E.

# 5

# Taking Care of You

So, how do you heal and repair your adrenals successfully? You might guess that lifestyle adjustments and dietary changes could make a difference. The issue, though, is that, as humans, we are likely to repeat our usual patterns, and we are drawn toward stress. Even with the best intentions, you may find yourself right back where you started: burned-out.

To pull yourself out of adrenal distress and prevent it from happening again, you need to figure out how to fit self-care into your daily routine. After talking and writing about diet, sleep, stress recovery, and exercise for years, I realized one day that it all fit into one healthy acronym: C.A.R.E.

In other words:

C: *Clean eating*
A: *Adequate sleep*
R: *Recovery*
E: *Exercise*

In the next few chapters, I'll help you implement my C.A.R.E. method based on your stress type, so you can maintain what you have discovered: your ability to respond and recover from stress in each moment and to be healthy, even while you're stressed. Changing your diet, sleep, stress levels, and exercise will—in conjunction with the Stress Recovery Protocol we'll cover in part three—heal your body from the inside out.

Before we dive in to understanding C.A.R.E. at a very deep level, I'd like to start with the big-picture view of how mastering stress fits into self-development and spiritual awakening.

## How to Shake Yourself Out of Stress Mode

Stress, of all types, causes us to go into survival mode. Our ego and fear keep us in survival mode (what I refer to as stress mode). From this perspective, we think we need to fight and struggle in order to survive each day. We look for and anticipate the next stress coming. In actuality, what we need is a release, a reset, to shift the pattern out of stress mode and into living authentically, powerfully, and freely. Our bodies know how to shift out of stress mode, just as a dog shakes off stress. The way our bodies do it is through shaking, vomiting, crying, singing, and yawning.

I observed and supported hundreds of women in labor—mainly home and birth-center births in the Seattle, Washington, area and hospital births in Manila in the Philippines. When observing women in labor, I noticed that they often shook, vomited, cried, and made sounds. That's also what my body did when I delivered my daughter at home. It is part of the process the body goes through when a person is in the middle of stress and pain.

Labor is a perfect example of harnessing stress. We need the stress response for labor to proceed, and we need support in order to prevent the stress from stopping labor. What I started to realize is that being human during regular daily life isn't that different. We need to learn to harness stress and our stress response by giving ourselves the right amount of support. It also means we need to allow our bodies to do what they naturally do to resolve stress—breathe, yawn, sing, moan, vomit, pee, poop, cry, and feel love and gratitude. It's in the rawness of being human and doing what humans do that stress recovery happens. If we resist and prevent ourselves from doing these fundamentally human activities, the stress remains, and it ends up causing other issues, blockages, and restrictions of energy and processes.

Here's what you need to do instead:

1.  Recognize that you are human and that you are loved and deserving.

2. Let go of identification with anything other than being human (a diagnosis, a title, or a role).
3. Allow yourself and your body to be in this moment, and trust that your body knows what it needs to recover from stress.
4. Accept support from loved ones, yourself, and your environment to harness the power of stress recovery.
5. Give your body the nutrients, food, water, rest, energy, and plants/herbs that it needs because it has been depleted by stress.

## Stand Back and Look at Your Life

It's one thing to work on stress recovery from within the framework and identity of our usual day-to-day lives. It's another thing to be able to step back and look at our lives and priorities, as well as our sense of self and purpose, from an outside perspective. Seldom do we have a chance to take such a big-picture look at our lives. Sometimes it happens when we are on vacation or traveling away from home. But often we are so caught up with the tasks at hand that we lose track of the days, months, and years. Next thing we know, life has passed us by.

I encourage you to create opportunities to take a break from your usual schedule and life so that you can look at things as an outsider would. Even if it's just for a long weekend. See if you can turn off your Wi-Fi and your cell phone. Step into a time and space where you don't have to make it to an appointment or meet a deadline. Sometimes we find ourselves creating alone-time without realizing that is what we are doing. It may just feel like you don't want to talk to anyone for a few hours or a few days. In those moments you can gain insights into why you do what you do and what you'd like to do differently going forward. I believe it is necessary for us to heal. In other words, it is our brain's way of creating the space to heal.

My grandmother was quite an inspiration to me. She was an unmarried teacher in a one-room schoolhouse when most women her age were married and did not work outside the home. She was independent and courageous like her mother, who ran a local restaurant in the small town in Oregon where they lived. Eventually my grandmother met and married my grandfather, who was ten years older. Together they ran a farm and business for several decades. At the age of fifty (which she reached at the end of World War II), my grandmother got in her car with her sister and girlfriend, and they drove all the way to Mexico City. My mother, then about six years old (and the youngest of three), stayed with my grandfather.

Why did my grandmother drive to Mexico City? Because she was tired of being home. She needed to get away, to get perspective on her life. To connect with herself. To understand her spirituality and her purpose.

She drove to Mexico City each year for several years. And then she decided it was time to go to Europe. She bought a bicycle, learned to ride it, and took a train across the country to New York. Then she took a flight to Europe, where she bicycled for weeks, from town to town, and country to country. She absolutely loved to travel and hoped to visit almost every country before she died. Many evenings, including the night she ended up passing away, I sat in her living room with her as she told me about the places and people she met in her travels.

She would say, "Always be willing to walk in another person's moccasins," a thought taken from a poem by Mary T. Lathrap. To me, this meant don't judge or criticize others—instead, be compassionate and learn from others. We can learn so much about ourselves from an outside perspective. We can also learn so much about ourselves when we get away from our usual day-to-day schedule and have a chance to reflect.

Much of what you'll learn in the following chapters will help you get a big-picture view of yourself, your life, and the way stress is affecting you. From that perspective, you'll have the opportunity to choose differently going forward in order to master your stress and reset your health.

## Why Is It So Hard to Care for Ourselves?

It tends to be so much easier to take care of others than to set aside time and resources to take care of ourselves. We're afraid of being told that we're selfish or self-centered, as if that's a bad thing. We have been taught to sacrifice ourselves and are rewarded for doing so. Denying ourselves what we need becomes so automatic. Even simple things like taking a shower or getting food for ourselves can seem unnatural. We are pros at taking care of others but not ourselves.

This is especially true if we are used to being dismissed or our needs have been neglected since childhood. We can feel as though we are not worthy or not enough, and this becomes a repeated pattern and self-fulfilling prophecy.

It's hard to know when we are stuck in this pattern, let alone how to break the cycle. It can seem impossible to let go of the fear and pain of the past—both physical and emotional. To do so requires a personal transformation, where we begin to feel that we are enough, that we are worth it and deserving of love simply because we exist.

We are so used to following a certain predetermined sequence each day of our lives: get up; get dressed and eat breakfast; brush our teeth; go to school or work; get married; have kids; and so on. We follow rules and aim to meet expectations. We worry that if we don't, we'll be alone, excluded, and unloved. We end up becoming less ourselves and more what we think we're supposed to be. Ultimately, we feel disconnected from our true selves, hopeless and helpless.

At that point, others don't know how to help, or they see our fear and pain and perhaps abandon us. Medically, people who reach this stage are diagnosed with a crisis, a breakdown, or psychosis. They are isolated and damped down with medications that mask emotional and physical pain.

But what if there was a way to break through instead of breaking down?

What if there was a way to shift or change our lives and the way we do and look at things without going through a crisis? What if that could be supported instead of judged? What if it could be a transformational experience?

I asked this (and wrote it) during the 2020 Covid-19 pandemic, while helping hundreds of patients under the greatest stress of their lives. Some—adults and teens—suffered such severe symptoms they went to a mental health institution and came out more traumatized. Others had tried taking medications for anxiety and grief and ended up with withdrawal symptoms and feeling as though they had lost their lives and themselves in the process. I saw single parents fearing whether they would be able to care for their children, and mothers and fathers who were stressed to the max about how to keep up and feel well enough to provide for their families. And I saw adults struggling to care for their aging parents in a world of new dangers.

This was also when I decided to go to Peru, where I spent three weeks with a shaman in the Sacred Valley, near Cusco. The experience forever shifted my perspective and ability to help myself and my patients. I was reminded that change is possible when we let go of the past. Things can work out differently in the future, even if we don't know exactly how or when. As the shaman said to me, enough is enough—perfection is stressful and impossible. We each have a gift or talent to share. Once we know our gift, it gives meaning and purpose to our lives.

We must tend to ourselves first. If you don't exist, nothing around you exists. If you are peaceful and joyful, everyone around you will be, too. If you are stressed, everyone will be stressed—it is contagious. You are not your body. You are not your emotions. You are not what happened to you. You are a unique being living in a human body with a human mind. The human nervous system is easily distracted and caught up in stress, so much so that we can lose track of our true selves. But we can reset from stress and find ourselves again.

Forgive yourself for whatever happened in the past. Accept and love yourself. That is something we can choose to do, and in doing so, we allow ourselves to heal.

Be grateful for your body—the three-dimensional vessel you live in. Take care of it and give value to it every day. By healing yourself, you give power to others to do the same. Stop fearing death and instead allow what *isn't* you (your distress) to die, so that you can live and die as your true self. You are enough. You are worthy and lovable because you are.

If we don't allow ourselves to do what humans do—cry, vomit, sleep, spit, poop, love, and feel connected—then we are not allowing ourselves to be fully human.

## What Is a Spiritual Transformation?

A spiritual connection to nature and self is transformational because it gives us an understanding of why we are here on this planet and what we are here to contribute. Having a sense of self—knowing oneself and loving oneself no matter what happened in one's past or what others have said or done—is often the beginning or first step in a spiritual transformation. By letting go of what has been said and unsaid, and choosing to connect with self anyway, we realize that we are who we were meant to be all along. We can learn to know what we need, how to receive it, and how to appreciate it.

From there, we can better connect with others and the world around us. This, by the way, is exactly how the Incas viewed life and spirituality more than five hundred years ago. They focused on understanding themselves, their purpose, and then the world and universe around them. They were great astronomers, without ever having a telescope.

I want to guide you to better become one with yourself.

To a place where being you feels natural and taking care of yourself feels automatic. Where you and your life are in sync. Where you wake up knowing you are in the right place at the right time. Where you are in such a state of alignment that you feel like you have become one with yourself and your experience. Like when you step into sand and your foot sinks in to mold and match the sand. Like when you go into water and the water flows around you. Like when you sink into your bed and the blankets wrap back around you.

To do this, you need to step back and connect with who you are. And to make choices to care for yourself through the food you eat, the activities you choose, the people you choose to be around, and the time you spend exercising, allowing your body to recover from stress, and resting or sleeping.

Before you learn how to do this, you need to pay attention to your spiritual self, in hopes of setting the foundation for real, honest change.

## Daily Spirituality

Spirituality begins with honoring aspects of nature that surround us and are essential for our existence on Earth, no matter our religion or faith. In naturopathic medical school, the curriculum includes courses in various systems of medicine, including Chinese medicine and Ayurvedic medicine. After taking these courses, I spent time learning from healers in Central America (Costa Rica, Nicaragua, and Mexico) and Asia (India, Japan, the Philippines, and Sri Lanka), as well as Spain, Turkey, Greece, Russia, and Iceland. Through these experiences, I came to understand the wisdom of medicine and spirituality in ancient cultures.

For example, in Chinese medicine, the parts of nature are referred to as "elements" and include earth, wood, fire, water, and metal. In Ayurvedic medicine, the elements are referred to as earth, fire, water, air/wind, and ether. Shamanism, from Tibet to South America, refers to the elements of earth, fire, water, and air.

These practices have in common a focus on supporting health for not just our bodies but our minds and spirits. If we don't give attention and support to understanding ourselves and our existence, then the lack of clarity can become a stress in itself that drives unwellness. For this reason, I've developed a layer within my Stress Recovery Protocol that gives you the opportunity to connect with yourself, with the people with whom you live and interact, and with the place you live on a spiritual level. The sense of gratitude and love that results can create an invisible scaffolding to support you and a safety net to catch you when stress becomes overwhelming.

Daily spirituality is integrated into the C.A.R.E. method in the form of acknowledging the aspects of nature we rely on, which become part of us and part of our existence. Without them, we would be nothing. In this way, they remind us of our humanness, the interconnectedness of all things, and the relative brevity of our opportunity to contribute to the world around us. We become humbled, letting go of our ego, which is what brings us to our knees in what is left: the spiritual realm.

## EARTH

Earth: Grounds us, provides stability and shelter. Rocks, dirt, sand, and mountains.

Wood: Provides shelter, strength, and calmness. Plants and trees.

## FIRE

Fire: Gives us heat, light, and energy; provides warmth and allows us to cook food and burn (or release) what we are no longer in need of. Flames and transformation of any sort.

## WATER

Water: Reminds us to flow, naturally and easily, and makes up 60 percent of our bodies. Ocean, rivers, lakes, rain, and tears.

## AIR

Wind: Provides air that we breathe and wind that is used for power and movement.

Ether or space: Creates the space we exist in and the sky, as well as the universe, unified field (quantum physics), and spiritual realm.

Metal: Represents breathing (lungs) and letting go of toxins (large intestines) and grief.

I will show you how to integrate these aspects of nature into your self-care routine, your environment, the foods you choose, and the nutrients and herbs (or plant medicines) used to support your stress recovery. By doing this, you will honor and appreciate yourself, the world around you, and you will also be better able to maintain a balance around you and within you.

6

# *C* for Clean Eating

The best way to think of clean eating is as a structure to eat what you need to support your health and stress recovery and to avoid the foods that can make matters worse. To help you get a better sense of what I mean by clean eating, I'll start with the basics of nutrition and continue on to describe ways of eating, foods to avoid, and foods to choose that will help you recover from stress, based on your stress type. Then, at the end of the book, I'll share my favorite recipes that integrate everything I describe about clean eating, so that you have a model to follow as you begin to make clean eating a priority in your life.

## Start with Basic Nutrition

Our food is composed of three main nutrients, referred to as macronutrients, which is where we get calories, glucose, amino acids, and fatty acids for our bodies to function and perform daily metabolism. Those three nutrients are protein, carbohydrates, and fats. When choosing the foods we eat, we should consider the relative quantity of protein, carbs, and fats in those foods.

When I was in college, studying nutrition, I was taught the standard nutritional guidelines according to the "Food Guide Pyramid" introduced by the

United States Department of Agriculture (USDA) in 1992. Those guidelines were developed at a time when medical practitioners were discouraging people from consuming more than 30 percent of calories from fats. Eating low fat or even "fat free" was promoted based on an unsubstantiated hypothesis that fat was associated with heart disease risk.[1] For that reason, the food pyramid emphasized getting the majority of our calories from carbohydrates, which included fruits, vegetables, and whole grains. When I analyzed this diet at the time, in the early 1990s, I found it impossible to follow without causing weight gain and blood sugar issues. I abandoned it myself and shifted to a diet with relatively equal parts of carbohydrates, protein, and fat.

More than twenty years later, in 2011, the USDA replaced the pyramid with "MyPlate," a graphic of a plate still showing "food groups" that call for a higher proportion of carbohydrates to other categories, even though research from 2006 demonstrated that a low-fat (increased carb) diet did not significantly reduce heart disease risk.[2] In 2019, with skyrocketing rates of diabetes and obesity, the American Diabetes Association finally released a statement acknowledging that lowering carbohydrate intake may improve blood sugar levels.[3] This is to say, beware of standard dietary recommendations. It's important to think them through for yourself and monitor how your body responds to any diet. You must decide for yourself how your body reacts to relative quantities of carbs, protein, and fats.

## Carbohydrates

Carbohydrates of all types, from cane sugar to carbs in vegetables and fruits, are broken down by our digestion to the smallest form, glucose, which is absorbed across the intestinal lining to enter our bloodstream. Insulin, a hormone made by the pancreas, is secreted and works to transport glucose from the blood into cells. Inside cells, glucose is used to make energy (carried in a molecule called ATP), which we use throughout our bodies for metabolic processes and muscle function. When insulin is working too well, or when we go too long between meals, we might experience a quick drop in blood sugar, known as hypoglycemia, which can cause irritability, nausea, and headaches. This is more likely for people with low cortisol levels, because their bodies may not be able to trigger a compensatory cortisol release when their blood sugar levels starts to drop, leaving them with low blood sugar.

When more glucose is consumed at one sitting than our body's insulin is able to move into cells, that extra glucose (referred to as blood glucose) is converted by the liver to either glycogen storage, cholesterol, or triglycerides; fat in the liver; or fat storage in the body (often around the waist).[4] Although scientists used to think that all cholesterol and body fat comes from fat in our diet, in actuality, it is the overeating of fats or carbs that cause the body to make more cholesterol. Once extra glucose is converted to fat, it is much harder for the metabolism to access it for use in making energy. It is more likely that the body will break down muscle tissue first.

The glycemic index indicates how quickly foods containing carbohydrate raise blood sugar levels. Processed sugar (white and brown sugar), for example, will raise blood sugar levels the fastest and highest, whereas vegetables and higher fiber grains tend be lower on the glycemic index. Fruits also vary in terms of the likelihood to raise glucose levels. Berries, cherries, grapefruit, and pears are the lowest.

I want to emphasize that while processed sugar (and processed food overall) is associated with higher risk of health issues (diabetes, heart disease, cancer, and dementia, to name a few), carbohydrates in general are essential.[5] The brain uses glucose to function, which is why our metabolism will prioritize the production of glucose from glycogen storage or by breaking down muscles when we are stressed. When cortisol becomes elevated with stress, this also increases blood glucose levels as a way to help us perform under pressure.

The problem arises when we are under chronic stress and cortisol remains elevated, such is the case for Stress Magnet, Night Owl, and Sluggish and Stressed stress types. In that situation, glucose levels remain high (hyperglycemia), even without consuming a high amount of carbs. Hyperglycemia leads to more inflammation and oxidative stress throughout the body (including the brain). It also causes weight gain, muscle loss, and cognitive decline.

While it's important not to overeat carbohydrates of any type, especially at one sitting, the goal is not to eliminate them completely, either. It's a matter of choosing the higher-fiber, less inflammatory types of carbs and include protein to prevent major blood sugar fluctuations. Carbohydrates from fruits and vegetables, particularly when eaten in digestible amounts and combined with healthy proteins and fats, contain antioxidants and improve methylation (use of B vitamins), while providing vitamins, minerals, and fiber. Grains are another source of carbohydrates that have been shown to be beneficial, in general, except for gluten-containing grains (barley, rye, spelt, and wheat), which are known to cause leaky gut and inflammation, especially in those who are genetically predisposed.[6] At the same time, it's possible to eat too much fruit, vegetables, and grains, increasing the risk of insulin resistance, high cholesterol, weight gain, imbalanced gut bacteria, and inflammation. Once again, enough is a good thing, and too much is what we are trying to avoid.

If you are concerned about your blood sugar levels, it can help to monitor your blood sugar levels for a period of time, say a week or two. You can purchase a glucose-monitoring device or ask your doctor to write a prescription for a continuous glucose-monitoring system. You'll want to know your fasting blood sugar when you wake in the morning and your blood sugar level two hours after eating. This way, you can look for patterns in terms of how much your blood sugar rises after eating certain foods and consuming certain quantities of food. It can be an eye-opening experience to actually see what your numbers are, and then to be able to proactively adjust your eating patterns to balance your blood sugar levels.

## Protein

Protein, which is broken down into amino acids in the digestive process, is used in the body for making muscles and neurotransmitters. Amino acids are also part of many metabolic processes, including detoxification and the production of antioxidants to protect cells from stress and inflammation. Protein also helps stabilize blood sugar levels, so if your blood sugar is dropping, eat protein.

Protein can be consumed in animal products—think beef, chicken, turkey, lamb, fish, eggs, and dairy products (cheese and yogurt)—as well as plant-based sources such as beans, nuts, seeds, and (in smaller quantities) grains and vegetables. Keep in mind that plant-based proteins come with carbohydrates and fats, whereas animal-based proteins do not contain substantial amounts of carbohydrates. Also, while animal-based protein sources are "complete proteins," meaning that they contain all nine amino acids essential for humans, plant-based proteins are not complete so they need to be eaten in combination with foods containing the other amino acids. This is why you'll often see beans combined with rice, for example.

Plant-based (vegan and vegetarian) diets have been studied many times and are strictly followed in areas of the world, such as India, where they accord with religious beliefs and are increasingly followed in the US, Europe, Israel, and Australia based on ethical or philosophical beliefs. Studies indicate a decreased incidence of heart disease (heart failure, in particular) and increased longevity with plant-based diets.[7] At the same time, plant-based diets are associated with a higher risk of anemia (due to low iron, B12, and folate) and nutrient deficiencies, and they can lead to imbalanced gut bacteria (bacterial overgrowth) when meal sizes are large.[8] While it is possible to successfully follow an entirely plant-based diet without experiencing deficiencies or other negative effects, it takes diligence and careful attention to ensure adequate nutrient and protein intake.

Higher-protein diets, including those based on plant-based protein, lead to improved body weight, greater exercise capacity, and increased muscle mass.[9] Studies estimate that consuming twenty-five to thirty grams of high-quality protein, in two or three meals per day, is necessary to stimulate muscle protein synthesis (MPS)—for making muscle—in healthy young and older adults.[10] As with almost everything, when protein intake becomes excessive, the benefit is lost (more is not better). It's a matter of consuming adequate protein from sources that work best for your body based on your stress type and activity level.

When cortisol levels are elevated for a long time, such as from chronic infection and for Stress Magnet and Sluggish and Stressed types, there is a loss of muscle (referred to as muscle wasting or cachexia). When I was recovering from adrenal distress, I found it imperative to include adequate protein at each meal, at consistent intervals each day. Without it, my blood sugar levels would vary, along with my energy level, mood, and sleep. I found that reaching for a variety of sources of protein works best for my body. I used both plant-based protein, such as pea protein for my shake and nuts/seeds in my muesli/granola, and fish/animal protein. As my adrenals recovered, I was able to be more reliant on plant-based protein, although when I have a busy schedule or am under stress, I do best with some animal protein each day.

## Fats

Healthy fats are needed for calories and for many other purposes in our bodies, including making hormones and cell walls. Fats also signal to the brain that we are full, so they increase satiety and help us feel that we have eaten. Fats also help decrease leptin, which can help with body weight. A low-fat diet is not recommended, although it is important to avoid certain types of fats that are oxidized or are in forms that our bodies can't use effectively. Avoid deep-fried fats and trans fats, which are manipulated chemically (as with margarine) and are known to increase inflammation in the body. Saturated fats, from meat and dairy products, are okay to some degree, but high amounts are associated with increased heart disease risk. Choose healthy fats such as olive oil (omega-9), flaxseed oil (omega-6), and fats in foods like olives, avocados, nuts, and seeds. Fish is also a great source of omega-3 fats.

A common misconception is that fats in our diet lead to fat in our blood vessels, such as cholesterol. In actuality, only a small percentage of fat from the diet turns into cholesterol. Instead, most cholesterol comes from the over-consumption of carbohydrates, which are turned into fats and cholesterol by the liver. The fats we consume are turned into hormones in our bodies, such as cortisol, DHEA, testosterone, estrogen, and progesterone. If your libido is low or you're having trouble getting pregnant, you may not be consuming enough fat in your diet.

At the same time, a high-fat diet, otherwise known as a ketogenic diet, is known to prevent and reverse diabetes and to assist with weight loss, and researchers are doing studies to see if it is helpful in addressing seizures, cancer, and dementia.[11] Meanwhile, cortisol and adrenaline tend to increase on a ketogenic diet (especially after exercising), which is an important consideration for Stress Magnet and Sluggish and Stressed types, who want to avoid pushing their levels even higher.[12] A ketogenic diet is 80 percent fats, with proteins and carbs kept to 10 percent each. Following a ketogenic diet, like other diets, requires a certain amount of preparation and planning, as well as monitoring ketone levels (in blood and/or urine), to get the most benefit from it.

A Mediterranean diet, on the other hand, is thought to be an example of a well-balanced diet. It is based on the traditional diet of people living in countries near the Mediterranean Sea, including France, Italy, Greece, and Spain. This way of eating includes carbs from vegetables, fruits, and whole grains; protein from fish and poultry as well as legumes and nuts; and fat from olive oil. The Mediterranean diet is associated with improved health and longevity, as well as decreased inflammation and more optimal cortisol levels.[13]

I've found a similar meal format in other parts of the world as well, such as Japan, India, the Philippines, and Central and South America. I believe this balanced way of eating is the most beneficial for healing adrenal distress for all the stress types, with slight tweaks, which I'll describe below. The general ratios to aim for are:

Protein: 20 to 40 percent of caloric intake
Carbohydrates: 15 to 30 percent of caloric intake
Fats: 25 to 40 percent of caloric intake

As you can see, a healthy diet is about having a balance of protein, carbo-hydrates, and fats, in their best forms and in quantities that suit your body's needs and patterns based on your stress type. Instead of just eating what's put in front of you, take charge of what you eat. Be purposeful about choosing what you put into your body.

## Eat Mindfully

"Mindful eating" involves devoting your full attention to the eating process, including how the food looks, tastes, feels, and smells. With each bite of food, you practice mindfulness, and you'll likely find a whole different eating expe-rience emerging. Most people report tasting their food as they never have before and feeling full faster. By focusing on chewing each bite, enjoying the food, and swallowing carefully, we send signals through our nervous system, and to the vagus nerve, to digest our food better; this signals to our brain that we have eaten.

So many signals occur when we eat. Hormones communicate to the pan-creas to release digestive enzymes and insulin. Hormones communicate to the brain to indicate hunger and fullness. Neurotransmitters and immune system signals communicate to the brain whether stress or inflammation is occurring in the digestion process. Gut bacteria also send signals to the immune and nervous systems. When we eat foods that are healthy for us and our microbi-ome, and we eat in a mindful way, the signals are calm and collected. When we eat in a stressed way, though, or when we eat foods that are more inflamma-tory or overfeed certain bacteria or other microbes, the signals shift to stress and inflammation.

The amount of food we eat at one sitting also has the potential to shift the signals we send to our digestion process. Eating just the right amount for our bodies, at a particular point in time, is what is needed to optimize communication. When we consume too much food, whether because we were taught to finish everything on our plates, or because the food tastes so good, or because we are distracted and not paying attention to each bite, all the signals shift to stress mode.

## Exploring Fasting

We use the word *fast* to indicate times when we're not eating. An overnight fast helps the digestion system reset. The most convenient and efficient means for doing this is while sleeping. In fact, it's why the first meal of the day is called *breakfast*, meaning "break the overnight fast."

There's a built-in motility and cleaning process called the migrating motor complex (MMC) that occurs three hours after a meal, and upon waking if we delay breakfast (not while we sleep). As soon as we eat, the MMC is turned off. Ideally, the MMC is able to clear out undigested food and toxin-producing bacteria, a process that takes one and a half to two hours.[14] This means we need to allow four and a half hours between meals and/or wait about two hours before eating our first meal of the day.

A recent trend called intermittent fasting emphasizes the overnight fast, and those following this practice may extend their overnight fast to fourteen or sixteen hours, delaying breakfast to late morning or noon, depending on when the last meal of the previous day occurred. While intermittent fasting is characterized by the length of the overnight fast, it is also focused on nutrient-dense and mindful meals during the eight-to-twelve-hour eating period. Intermittent fasting has been shown to improve MMC function (and digestion overall), improve insulin function (it increases the responsiveness of cells' insulin, therefore decreasing blood sugar levels), decrease body fat, and support mitochondrial function (energy production) and autophagy (clean out cells).[15] It also increases cortisol levels, which may be desired for Blah and Blue and Tired and Wired types who wake up with low cortisol.[16]

As with most practices, it's possible to overdo intermittent fasting. It needs to be modified based on your stress type, blood sugar levels, digestion, and daily routine. If you fast for too long, it can actually cause cortisol levels to increase too much and trigger a stress response; this works against your original intention, especially if you are a Stress Magnet or Sluggish and Stressed type.[17] In a process similar to what happens with an eating disorder, your body can go into starvation mode, disrupting cortisol levels and causing them to increase. Then, when you do eat, calories tend to be stored, causing weight gain and potentially leading to a vicious cycle of abstaining and gaining. Conversely, if you consume too large of a meal because you're overly hungry, you're likely to not digest it well, thus overfeeding gut bacteria and causing gas and bloating.

I often joke that I wish our bodies came a with a clear signal—a flashing light, for example—to tell us when we need to eat and when we've eaten enough. Instead, you have to try out varying amounts of food and different mealtimes to find what works best for you, based on your stress type and where you are in the Stress Recovery Protocol. Blah and Blue and Sluggish and Stressed, who are more likely to have hypoglycemia or low blood sugar levels, may need to eat a little more often to prevent a roller-coaster ride of blood sugar levels. As cortisol and adrenaline come closer to optimal, these types will be able to go longer between meals without sending out stress signals.

Here's one way to think about designing a food plan. First, imagine all the food you would eat in one day. Then split it into four sections, each with adequate protein and healthy fats. Those are your four meals for the day. Now all you need to do is eat them a few hours apart.

If you tend to eat more than needed at each sitting and end up too full or bloated, try reducing your meals by two bites (two bites of carbs, preferably); in other words, leave two spoonfuls on the plate and/or put them in the fridge for later. Do this for each meal of the day and I think you'll find that you won't miss those bites at all. At the same time, the total reduction in excess calories and carbs will make a big difference for your body in terms of decreased stress and inflammation. Another idea is to serve your meal on a smaller plate or in a smaller bowl. I serve all my meals on salad plates and in small soup bowls. I also eat with a small fork. All of these choices help me eat the amount of food I know my body can effectively digest, absorb, and metabolize.

So here, again, the message is to listen to your body, know your stress type, and make modifications to get the most positive, healthful effect possible without pushing it too far in one direction or another. We need to be mindful that as humans we tend to want to "push through," be competitive, be perfectionistic, exceed expectations, and impress. Yet those tendencies can also lead us into stress mode, even when doing something "healthy." So be careful! When applying the concept of hormesis to dietary changes and fasting, the goal is to make just enough change to bring your cortisol, blood sugar levels, and body to an optimal balance, but not too much or too extreme, which would be stressful and potentially damaging.

Another form of fasting called a fasting-mimicking diet (FMD) is an example of hormesis and adapted homeostasis. Fasting-mimicking has been studied as a way to get the benefits of fasting while still eating,[18] by consuming a very specific amount of carbohydrates, protein, and fat that turns off certain metabolic pathways in the body, enabling the body to clean out cells (autophagy) and reset, literally, at a cellular level, to allow for improved insulin function and increased longevity. This diet is based on systems of fasting that have been used over centuries and in many religions. In particular, this diet has been used by people who live in "blue zones," which are parts of the world where people live the longest. The fasting-mimicking diet is implemented for five days at a time and can be repeated for three months in a row, and then every three to four months, for the greatest benefit. It is through restricting our diet in such a way that we also increase our mindfulness and appreciation for our food.

When I first followed the fasting-mimicking diet, I found it interesting that it allows you to eat several small meals throughout the day but results in an overall decrease in calories. It also involves a higher intake of carbs and a lower amount of protein than I'm accustomed to eating. However, this is the shift that is needed for the positive effect to occur. As with any health practice, it's important to know your body when following this diet. For instance, if you have kidney or liver disease, or if you're currently at the extreme end of stress mode, this isn't a good time to try this way of eating. Stabilize your body first by following a diet that decreases stress messages. Once you're out of stress mode, then you can implement a fasting-mimicking and/or intermittent fasting diet plan. By doing things in this order, you'll avoid making your health worse.

Please keep in mind that fasting for extended periods of time, or for more than twenty-four hours, leads to an increase in cortisol in the morning and throughout the day. I've seen these curves in patients of mine when they were either recovering from anorexia or dealing with severe stress and digestive issues. Multiple days of fasting are rarely recommended, especially if you are already under stress or if you are a Stress Magnet. It's important to avoid going beyond the beneficial period, or what we call the hormetic zone, and avoid stressing your body even more by using extreme fasting techniques. Even when I had severe headaches caused by neck muscle spasms and associated vomiting for twelve to twenty-four hours, as soon as I possibly could, I would get back to eating. I'd start with the smallest possible quantity of cooked and easily digested foods and continue until my digestion was ready for more regular meals.

## Eating Clean Means Minding the Details

Above all else, be sure to avoid processed foods. When foods are premade, packaged, and sold at the store, often other ingredients are added to improve the taste, texture, and freshness. This means that along with the food, you are getting chemicals that can potentially send stress signals to your gut, nervous system, hormones, and immune system. Check the label on the package for any additives that you don't want to eat. Best of all is to buy the actual foods and make your meals yourself, so that you know exactly what the ingredients are. In my family, we've even started making our own ice cream so that we can use the type of milk (nondairy) and sweetener (maple syrup) we prefer and avoid all the gums and other ingredients we don't want. If you don't like to cook, consider ordering from a meal delivery service that offers dairy-free, gluten-free, and sugar-free options. The term *paleo* is often used to describe food that meets these criteria.

Choose organic, as well. Each spring, the Environmental Working Group releases its "dirty dozen" and "clean fifteen" produce lists. Certain fruits and vegetables are known to have high amounts of pesticide exposure. Absolutely aim to buy organic when it comes to foods on the "dirty dozen" list. The "clean fifteen" are the foods that tend to have the lowest levels of pesticides. Still, my rule of thumb is to buy organic as often as possible, or always. I also shop for "pasture-raised," "grass-fed" meats that have not been exposed to antibiotics and are organic whenever possible. It can be hard to find restaurants that pay attention to avoiding toxins in their food, but I have discovered and enjoyed some amazing organic eateries and have found businesses offering clean options on their menus.

Decreasing or avoiding sugar, especially in the form of actual cane sugar, as in white and brown sugar, is also important. Often sugar will be replaced in products with coconut palm sugar or monk fruit, which is a better option because it offers sweetness but is less likely to raise blood sugar levels. The preferred option, however, is stevia because it comes from a plant and tastes sweet, but doesn't trigger an insulin response—this means it also doesn't increase risk of diabetes or inflammation. Sugar, on the other hand, is known to raise blood sugar levels, overwhelm insulin function, increase cholesterol levels, and raise inflammation while decreasing immune function and leaving us vulnerable to all sorts of health issues.

The amount of sugar in foods quickly adds up, between packaged and baked goods, and beverages and even condiments. Before you know it, you could be consuming way more sugar than you even realize. Start by checking labels and decreasing the use of sugar in recipes. Often the same recipe tastes just as good or better without sugar. Fructose, which is the sugar found in fruit, honey, and maple syrup, is another option that's healthier than other sugars, but it's still important to be careful of the quantities here, because fructose can overfeed gut bacteria and yeast, and can stress the liver, too.[19] High fructose corn syrup (HFCS) is a sweetener used in packaged foods and is best avoided because it is linked to diabetes and fatty liver.

Decrease or avoid caffeine while clean eating, since it is known to increase both cortisol and adrenaline levels.[20] Depending on your stress type, you may currently be relying on caffeine to get you through the day. Stopping cold turkey isn't the best option then. Instead, the goal is to help your body recover from stress. As your cortisol and adrenaline levels stabilize and improve on their own, you'll become less reliant on caffeine for energy.

Decrease or avoid alcohol, too, as it must be metabolized by the liver, which makes it a stress to your body and means that your body will require antioxidants to help it recover. Plus, drinking alcohol is associated with a rise in dopamine followed by a dip, which, along with the dehydration it causes, leads to a hangover; this is your body's way of telling you that it's stressed and needs to recover. Studies show that a low intake of alcoholic drinks is okay and that the resveratrol in red wine is particularly protective.[21] So, if you choose to have red wine (which I do every so often), choose biodynamic, organic wines without additives or sulfites. Women should drink no more than one glass of wine in one day and no more than four glasses per week. Men should drink no more than two glasses of wine in one day and no more than six glasses per week. It's also possible to get resveratrol from berries and supplements, so you don't have to miss out on it if you abstain from alcohol.

Choose foods high in antioxidants and related phytochemicals, which exist in herbs, fruits, and veggies. When in doubt, turn to color, as antioxidants give foods their beautiful hues. Think of green, purple, orange, red, blue, yellow, and even white options when choosing fruits and veggies. For example, tomatoes, papaya, and watermelon contain lycopene, which is known to decrease heart disease risk. These plant substances help us recover from stress and trauma by protecting cells. My favorites are wild, organic blueberries; broccoli; and leafy greens, such as kale, arugula, and chard. Then there is chocolate! Cocoa beans (which are used to make chocolate) are high in antioxidants and have been shown to be beneficial to our health.[22] Just be sure to choose dark chocolate (at least 70 percent cocoa) and avoid products with added sugar.

When eating clean, choose foods to support liver detoxification, such as root vegetables like sweet potatoes, turnips, and carrots; artichokes; leafy greens; and cruciferous vegetables like broccoli, brussels sprouts, and cauliflower. They all contain substances that assist with detoxification pathways.

## Eating Clean by Decreasing Inflammation

Avoiding foods that increase inflammation is of utmost importance when clean eating. Sugar is one of the most important to watch out for. Other inflammatory foods include dairy products (foods made from cow milk) and gluten (wheat, rye, spelt, barley). In some cases, the food reaction is caused by not digesting the food or component of the food well. Other times it is due to a specific protein in the food triggering an immune response.

Dairy is a perfect example. When people are lactose intolerant, it is because they are not digesting the sugar in milk products well. They are likely to experience bloating and digestive issues. Alternatively, when people react to the proteins in milk, casein and whey, it causes an inflammatory response that can spread throughout the body, and is associated with sinus congestion, ear infections, anxiety, and more. Grains containing gluten are most likely to increase inflammation and to cause leaky gut, making it more likely you'll react to additional foods. People with severe leaky gut are more likely to react to grains that don't contain gluten, such as rice, millet, corn, and oats, as well as nuts and seeds.

The inflammation can be due to an antibody response—an outright allergy (IgE antibodies) or a delayed food sensitivity (mediated by IgA and

IgG antibodies). For others, it may be due to a histamine release, which can be influenced by genetics, imbalanced gut bacteria, and/or mold toxicity.[23] It is also possible to react due to salicylates, oxalates, or sulfur in the food, and/or to foods that are nightshades. Or it could be due to all of the above, in which case it can begin to seem like almost every food is inflammatory, which is a sure sign of leaky gut and imbalanced gut bacteria.

Foods that trigger histamine responses include citrus fruits, tomatoes, bananas, spinach, avocado, chocolate, nuts, wheat, alcohol, fermented foods, and aged meats and cheese. Salicylates are high in almonds, apples, apricots, berries, cherries, cucumbers, and grapes/raisins. Oxalates are high in leafy greens, beets, nuts, berries, chocolate, and wheat. Sulfur is high in garlic, onions, chicken, cruciferous vegetables (broccoli, brussels sprouts), artichokes, asparagus, beans, chocolate, coffee, and eggs (among others). Nightshades include potatoes, tomatoes, eggplant, and peppers. If you notice you are reacting to these foods, decrease your exposure while you work on healing leaky gut.

You can imagine that reacting to all these different factors would greatly limit your diet. Once again, I want to warn you to be careful of extreme dietary restrictions, which can become more of a stress than the stress you're trying to solve in the first place. *Orthorexia* is a term used to describe an unhealthy restriction of food due to taking clean eating to an extreme. Working with a practitioner who is highly skilled in clinical nutrition will make all the difference for you in ensuring that you get enough calories and nutrients, while avoiding reactions as much as possible and giving your body the support it needs to heal.

One way to approach avoidance of inflammatory foods is by following a food elimination diet.[24] This type of diet involves avoiding the most common (or most likely) inflammatory foods—often that would be dairy, gluten, eggs, soy, and nuts—for at least twenty-one days. Then the foods are reintroduced, one by one, with three or four days in between to observe for reactions. While a food elimination diet is considered a standard approach, from my experience it is limited in that the whole process can take over a month and is dependent on being able to notice that you react to a food when you bring it back into your diet.

I find it to be more efficient to do a highly sensitive IgA and IgG antibody food panel, as described in chapter four, and then eliminate the highest reactive foods. By doing it this way, you don't have to guess which foods are inflammatory—the results show you—and you can get right to avoiding the foods that are making the leaky gut worse.

I've been guiding patients through this process for over twenty years, and I went through it myself, which is why I know it's possible to achieve great health while following my eating plans. The key is to eat your safest (least reactive) foods, prepare your meals at home, eat at regular intervals throughout the day, include protein and healthy fats, and follow my protocol to heal leaky gut in chapter ten.

## Feeding Your Microbiome

Choosing foods to feed (but not overfeed) good bacteria is an absolute must. The types and quantities of bacteria living in our intestines are determined by what we eat. They feed off fiber, which we don't digest or absorb. Any other undigested food also feeds the bacteria, so when we are under stress and not digesting well, a lot of what we eat feeds the bacteria instead of feeding us. To feed the bacteria most likely to support our health, we need to consume what are referred to as resistant starches. That's because resistant starches are fermented into short-chain fatty acids to feed colon cells and increase regulatory T (Treg) cells in the immune system, which are known to decrease allergies, asthma, and autoimmunity. When we are stressed or exposed to trauma, it decreases Treg cells, which makes us vulnerable to health issues, including leaky gut and inflammation. The foods containing the most resistant starch are leeks, onions, asparagus, and garlic.

Prebiotics (otherwise known as food for good bacteria), such as fructooligosaccharides (FOS) and Bimuno galacto-oligosaccharides (B-GOS), lower the cortisol awakening response, indicating that they can potentially modulate the HPA axis and be especially helpful for Stress Magnets and Sluggish and Stressed types.[25] No matter what your stress type, feeding our gut bacteria the right fibers/starches helps us recover from stress. This includes fiber from berries, nuts, seeds, vegetables, and fruits. At the same time, be careful not to overdo it, because overfeeding the bacteria can have the opposite response. You don't have to consume huge quantities to benefit your good bacteria. Even a teaspoon of ground flaxseeds or a quarter cup of frozen blueberries will be plenty to feed your bacteria.

Too often, I hear from patients who have been overdoing green smoothies by adding three cups of leafy greens to a cup of fruit. We simply can't digest that much food at once, and it's way more than our bacteria need at a single serving, too. What can end up happening is small intestinal bacterial overgrowth (SIBO), which occurs when the bacteria in the small intestine are essentially having a party at our expense, leaving us bloated, burping, and in pain. The same can happen when we overconsume fermented foods, which are a wonderful idea, just not in large quantities. If we add too many bacteria to our digestion, even good bacteria can cause trouble.

At that point, when addressing overgrowing bacteria, it can be helpful to follow what is called the FODMAP diet, which stands for fermentable oligosaccharides, disaccharides, monosaccharides, and polyols (sugar alcohols). The FODMAP diet was designed to help people with fructose intolerance, which is a decreased ability to digest fructose, whether due to genetic causes or a leaky gut. You see, one of the jobs of the small intestinal cells is to digest fructose; however, with leaky gut, there are fewer cells to perform this role, so fructose is left undigested. When this occurs, the bacteria love it, because they have more food for themselves, leading to yet more bloating and gas. Whether you're experiencing bloating due to fructose intolerance, SIBO, or both, following a diet that is low in fructose and other similar starches is going to decrease your symptoms and make it harder for the bacteria to flourish quite so much.

## Spirituality of Food

More than anything, I want to emphasize the opportunity to honor the food you eat as it nourishes you on many levels. You may find it helps to think of food in terms of the four elements—earth, fire, water, and air. The goal is to choose foods to balance your body.

Earth: Choose sweet and starchy foods, including root vegetables and soft fruits—millet, oats, cooked onion, watermelon, sweet apples, sweet cherries, dates, grapes, peaches, carrots, cabbage, potatoes, sweet potatoes, yams, bananas, cucumbers, beets, mushrooms, almonds, coconuts, papayas, lentils, peas, honey, and maple syrup—as well as hearty meats like beef. The wood aspect of earth includes sour foods, such as citrus fruits, pineapple, vinegar, yogurt, and olives; and foods with stalks or sprouts, such as bok choy, spinach, chard, broccoli, asparagus, and celery.

**Fire:** Choose bitter foods, red and heart-shaped foods, dry and hot foods, lamb, lettuce, arugula, tomatoes, apricots, citrus peel, plums, raspberries, strawberries, peppers, paprika, and chocolate.

**Water:** Choose salty and dark-colored foods, filtered water, root vegetables, seaweed and seafood, eggs, soy sauce and tamari, blueberries and blackberries, eggplant and kale, walnuts, and sesame, sunflower, and pumpkin seeds.

**Air:** Choose savory and pungent foods and white foods, such as mushrooms, rice, raw onion, garlic, chives, radishes, cauliflower, tofu, pears, cinnamon, mint, tarragon, marjoram, rosemary, thyme, cloves, fennel, cilantro, coriander, anise, dill, basil, mustard greens, horseradish, and nutmeg.

Aim to include each of these elements each day and each time you create a meal. You'll find examples of this in the recipes I have provided at the end of the book. In this way, you direct your attention away from stressing about food and toward appreciation for your body and for nature, which provides what we need to survive and thrive.

## Following a Stress Reset Cleanse

When you're able to set aside time for a full stress reset in the form of a five- or ten-day retreat or escape from your usual life and stress exposure, including a break from Wi-Fi and cell service and a chance to spend time in nature and with yourself, then you can follow a diet intended to induce deeper healing. This is the perfect way to reset your autonomic nervous system, HPA axis, and support autophagy at the same time.

When working with the shaman in Peru, for example, for ten days I followed a strict *dieta* of no sugar, no salt, no meat or fish, no dairy, no gluten, and no caffeine, alcohol, or chocolate. I also disconnected from Wi-Fi and my cell phone, spent time in nature every day, and fasted overnight for twelve to sixteen hours. I was also able to focus on eating mindfully and experiencing food spiritually.

Going into it, I wasn't sure how I would feel, but I was pleased to find that the *dieta* matched up very well with my goals of de-stressing and realigning with my circadian rhythm. This is to say that there is value in following a cleanse or diet for short periods of time as a sort of stress reset and healing support process, but I always suggest working with a practitioner who can help assess your adrenal function and overall health to help prepare you and support you. Better yet is a stress reset based on your stress type! That is how I guide participants in my programs.

## Eating for Your Stress Type

### Stress Magnet

Your days are packed with activities, and you are aware of your own tendency to put your business ahead of your own needs. Therefore, you should prepare food ahead of time and have it available to grab every three to five hours to reduce the temptation to skip meals. Because your cortisol and adrenaline levels are already high, it's important for you to avoid extreme fasting, intermittent fasting, and even a ketogenic diet until after you get your body out of stress mode. Stick to meals that contain a slightly higher percentage of protein, along with low glycemic carbs, and fat, at regular intervals throughout the day to give your body the signal that stress has subsided and that it's safe to bring your cortisol and adrenaline back to optimal levels. Caffeine, sugar, and alcohol will only work against you. At the same time, prebiotics can work for you by helping to prevent a cortisol spike in the morning.

### Night Owl

You might add a second, small dinner containing carbs and protein to your meal plan to keep from snacking on popcorn or ice cream late at night while finishing up a report or catching up on laundry. Food cravings and high-carb snacks will only further disrupt your blood sugar, cortisol, and sleep patterns. Stay in front of cravings by planning ahead and eating half-sized meals throughout the day and up to about three hours before bed. Then stop eating and give yourself an intermittent fast until morning. This will help reset your circadian rhythm. If you absolutely need to eat something in order to get to sleep, then choose protein—a protein shake is perfect here. Stay away from sugar, which will only perpetuate the unwanted pattern.

## Sluggish and Stressed

With your combination of high cortisol and low adrenaline, it's best for you to avoid extreme diet plans, fasting, or calorie restriction. Stick to meals that contain a consistent amount of carbs, protein, and fat at regular intervals throughout the day and stop eating about three hours before bed. Morning is especially important for you because it gives you a chance to reset your stress pattern. Make sure to create a calm morning experience, with stress recovery activities (which I'll cover in chapter 8), and don't fast for too long; you'll likely do better with a meal containing protein and carbs soon after you wake. Delay caffeine for an hour or so if possible, and keep it to a minimum to allow your adrenals to recover. As your system calms down and comes out of stress mode, you'll be able to support your energy with real adrenaline, so aim for that rather than temporary adrenaline boosts.

## Blah and Blue

At first, you might need to eat in smaller amounts more often, every two hours or so, to improve your energy and blood sugar levels. That's because when cortisol and adrenaline are low, you'll tend to have hypoglycemia, or dips in your blood sugar levels, even when you're not eating sugar, due to your adrenal glands' inability to effectively manage your blood sugar levels. This means you have to manage them with carefully planned, protein-rich meals. With consistency and adrenal healing, you'll soon find that you can space your meals out a bit more without triggering hypoglycemia. You may also initially find that you need a little caffeine to help you through your day, which is okay for your stress type while you heal. Just don't overdo it and send yourself into an overstimulated state. It's likely that a relatively low-carb diet, higher in protein and fat, or even a ketogenic diet, may help your energy and mood. That's because it will help give you energy. Just remember to take it easy and listen to your body.

## Tired and Wired

You have the low cortisol of Blah and Blue but the high adrenaline of a Stress Magnet, which means you'll apply a bit from both of those stress types to your eating plan. In your case, delaying breakfast to create a little bit longer intermittent fast could help increase your cortisol. Then, when you're ready to eat, you'll probably feel best with a protein shake before too much time passes; what's more, you should stay away from caffeine as it will raise your adrenaline. Eat a small meal containing protein every three to five hours, depending on how stable your blood sugar levels are and how much time you feel you need to allow the MMC to help heal your digestion. Follow a lower-carb, higher-protein diet to help bring your cortisol levels up and your adrenaline down.

# 7

# *A* for Adequate Sleep

don't know about you, but I grew up thinking that sleep wasn't so important. "I'll sleep when I die" and "I don't have time to sleep" were common
expressions I'd hear all the time. In some ways, I'm grateful that my parents
didn't stress about bedtime. At the same time, I often went to bed late and
woke up early in order to be ready to head out the door to go to school, to go
skiing or hiking, or to attend some other activity. I was also afraid of the dark
and had nightmares, so I often slept with the light on and woke up several
times each night (now I know how detrimental that was to my health).

When my daughter was young, she had a hard time falling asleep and
would wake up throughout the night, too. That meant I didn't get much sleep
for several years, until she started sleeping better. I think that, as parents,
we downplay sleep because we have to prioritize taking care of our kids.
Nonetheless, it quickly became apparent that even when my daughter was
sleeping, I stayed up working on patient charts or writing, thinking it was
more important for me to get more done in a day than to sleep. It was only
when I wrote a book on natural solutions to insomnia that I convinced myself
to prioritize sleep.

I resolved that I would not publish the insomnia book until I was getting at least seven and a half hours of sleep each night! In doing so, I came to really understand the difference it makes to get good sleep.

The truth is that so much restoration occurs in our bodies when we sleep. Ideally, our cortisol levels drop to give our body a break and then increase when we wake, giving us energy to start our day. It's important for our bodies to experience hours when cortisol is low, and we need the adrenal reset overnight to achieve that. I suggest at least seven and a half hours of sleep to support your adrenals, with nine hours being ideal, as often as possible. Changes in our sleep pattern disrupt our cortisol levels, and sleep deprivation activates a stress response, both of which are associated with increased risk of diabetes, cancer, decreased memory, and depression.[1]

You want as much as possible of the sleep you get to be uninterrupted. You may even have to plan for it, scheduling sleep with the same level of prioritization you would an important meeting. At the same time, I'm going to show you how you can prevent lack of sleep from negatively affecting your health. In this chapter, I'll review why sleep matters, plus discuss how much is enough and how to improve your sleep based on your stress type.

## What We Know About Sleep

You're not alone in your struggles with sleep. In 2014, the Centers for Disease Control and Prevention declared sleep deprivation to be a public health epidemic. Imagine! An epidemic! Plus, my own patients always tell me how much they struggle with sleep. And I understand that reading about how important sleep is can trigger you to feel stressed about not sleeping as much as you should. Before we dive in to understanding sleep, I really want to encourage you to be gentle with yourself. Instead of fighting against, or thinking negative thoughts about, your body for keeping you awake, focus on what your body is signaling to you. What can you do to help your body get better sleep?

Addressing sleep, after all, offers the perfect chance to realize that it doesn't help to stress more about stress (or stress about a lack of sleep). That just leads to fewer hours of rest! Shift your mind to a place of curiosity, not self-judgment, and know that things can improve.

Sleep is composed of distinct stages that repeatedly cycle. The stages are essentially like stairsteps or shifting gears from awake to deep sleep. Deep sleep is considered stage three or four (it is called by different names in the research). Our brain waves change at each stage of sleep, with slow-wave oscillations, referred to as delta brain waves, occurring at the deepest levels. After deep sleep, we bounce back to stage two and then transition to rapid eye movement (REM) sleep. It takes about ninety minutes to cycle through these stages, and with each cycle, more time is spent in REM sleep, starting with ten minutes in the first cycle.

When thinking about and researching sleep, scientists look at sleep quality, duration, and timing. Quality has to do with how quickly we fall asleep, whether we wake at night, and how often we wake. Optimally, we fall asleep within twenty minutes. Sleep duration is how long we sleep. Less than seven hours per twenty-four-hour period is considered to be too little sleep.

Sleep timing has to do with how our hours of sleep line up with a healthy circadian rhythm. Our circadian rhythm determines when we are awake and when we sleep based on light and darkness, otherwise known as the sleep-wake cycle. We want the midpoint of sleep to be between midnight and 3 AM because those are the hours when deep sleep is most likely to happen in the circadian rhythm. If we go to sleep after 1 AM, we'll get less deep sleep because we'll have only two hours to get in our deep sleep, and a whole sleep cycle lasts ninety minutes, so we'll run out of time for more. Another way to look at this is that we want to get the most deep sleep as possible in the first four hours of our sleep period, and then we want REM sleep to take up most of the last four hours of our sleep.

Deep sleep should account for 15 to 25 percent of your total sleep time. Optimally, REM sleep should be 20 to 25 percent of your total sleep in the final stage before you wake in the morning. Deep sleep is the most difficult to wake up from, even when there are loud noises. If you are woken from a deep sleep, you're more likely to experience brain fog for thirty to sixty minutes. If you are used to sleeping four to five hours each night, as you adjust to sleeping more, you might actually feel groggier at first. That's because you might be reaching deep sleep, instead of REM sleep, right before you wake up.

Both deep sleep and REM sleep decrease with age. While infants spend eight hours a day in REM, seventy-year-olds spend only forty-five minutes in REM. It's not that we don't need sleep as we get older. We do! It's that we are less capable of getting good sleep as we age, and the lack of sleep predisposes us to health issues. Sleep disorders, for example, are prevalent in neurodegenerative disease and dementia. This means that lack of sleep increases risk, and neurodegenerative disorders often cause sleep disruption. Sleep deprivation has also been linked to cardiovascular disease, high blood pressure, diabetes, excess body weight, and preventable accidents.

Finally, sleep deprivation is associated with higher cortisol levels and a greater increase in cortisol when exposed to stress.[2] Elevated cortisol becomes a vicious cycle: high cortisol disrupts sleep, and a lack of sleep causes cortisol to go higher. Waking up after sleeping part of the night is also associated with an increase in adrenaline.[3] Naps, on the other hand, help us recover from a lack of sleep. A study showed that cortisol levels reset during a two-hour nap.[4]

## Our Bodies Love to Sleep

A lot of good stuff happens when we sleep. For one, melatonin, known as our sleep hormone, increases when our brains perceive darkness. You want to sleep in a dark room—and the darker it is, the better for your melatonin production. Studies are showing that melatonin not only is important for signaling our bodies to sleep but also plays a role as an antioxidant and in the immune system by protecting us from infections and cancer.[5] Melatonin is made in the pineal gland from serotonin, so if you're low on serotonin, your body may not have enough of the precursor nutrients and amino acids to make melatonin. Light exposure, especially at night, also deceases melatonin production.

Melatonin also signals to the hypothalamus to increase the production of growth hormone by the pituitary gland. Growth hormone, which helps with repair and regrowth of muscles and bones, is also important for immune function and is secreted only during deep sleep. Growth hormone counteracts the pitfalls of aging, so to prevent aging, we need more sleep! And a lack of sleep is a major stress on our bodies. The more deep sleep we get, the better.

In 2012, the glymphatic system, which is the brain's built-in waste clearance system, was discovered. It eliminates proteins and metabolites from the central nervous system and is active only during deep sleep.[6] If we don't get deep sleep, we are more prone to building up amyloid and tau proteins, which are associated with dementia. Studies have shown that getting more deep sleep slows the progression of neurodegenerative disease.[7]

Weight gain, which aggravates sleep issues, is also caused by lack of sleep for several reasons, one of which involves two hormones related to hunger: ghrelin and leptin. When we are deprived of sleep, ghrelin increases and leptin decreases, stimulating appetite and causing us to eat more.[8] Another reason is that cortisol increases when we don't sleep well, decreasing our ability to manage glucose.[9] Additionally, endocannabinoids, which I'll discuss in chapter 8, increase when we don't get enough sleep, and they increase cravings for sweets and carbs, which makes matters worse. As weight increases, the risk of sleep apnea also increases.

## How to Track Your Sleep

It has become easy and popular to track your sleep using a device and/or an app on your smartphone. This can be a great way to learn more about your sleep patterns and to know where you are starting from. As you make changes to your diet, stress levels, and exercise routines, you can monitor your sleep patterns and see what's making a difference and how.

For example, there are finger rings, wristbands, headbands, and even sleep pads that can monitor your sleep when you bring them to bed. They can show sleep timing and patterns, such as how much time you spend in deep sleep. In some cases, these devices rely on Bluetooth or Wi-Fi, so if you want to keep technology out of your bedroom or find yourself looking at your phone screen too often, try using the device or app for a couple of days to establish a starting point. Then move your phone out of the bedroom. After you feel some improvement has been made, take another reading for a day or two to see your progress.

## Sleep Hygiene and Your Sensory System

There are several practices you can incorporate into your daily routine to improve your sleep quality and duration. These practices are referred to as sleep hygiene. Believe it or not, your behaviors throughout the day, especially before bedtime, have a major impact on your ability to sleep well. This means that everything from your sleep environment to the very bed you sleep on can be a factor in determining your sleep cycles. Even with your eyes closed, all five of your senses are processing and delivering information to your brain, and in turn affecting sleep quality.

Your five senses influence, and are influenced by, your sleep patterns. Let's break each one down.

## Sight

Walk into your bedroom and do a 360-degree scan. What do you see? If the place you begin and end your day feels scattered and all over the place, likely you will, too. Several studies have reported that a cluttered bedroom can have a negative impact on your sleep and overall well-being. So ask yourself if you feel calm and serene in this space. If you don't, what is it that's bothering you? Are there piles waiting for you? Does it appear as though the Tasmanian Devil just ran through your closet, leaving a trail of clean and dirty clothes strewn across the floor? It's amazing how our perception of our space, the literal to-do list in our visual field, can influence our mental state and ability to sleep. It's time to create the Zen zone your body and mind needs.

Stop your space from working as more than your bedroom. If you're working from home, you may find that the distinction between relaxation and work is slipping. It's okay, because this happens even without a work-from-home mandate, but let's change this. If you have the option, make your bedroom a place that is naturally associated with rest and relaxation. This will immediately change your environment and your mindset. Then, when you lie down in bed, your body and brain will know that this is where you can decompress.

Surveys have found that neutral, muted shades of blue, yellow, silver, and green are the most relaxing color palettes for a sleep environment. If you have vibrant paint on your walls or patterns on your bedding that are highly stimulating, consider swapping them out for something more relaxing. Another easy and highly effective fix is to adorn your windows with blinds and/or drapes to make sure that your room stays dark throughout your sleep. I recommend blackout shades to ensure that you can eliminate light while you sleep.

Most of us start and end our day the same way, with our phone in hand and staring at a screen. And depending on our work environment, the middle portion of our day isn't much different. While all this tech has brought many wonderful things to our lives, it also has a tremendous effect on our health. Our brains pick up on the artificial blue light emitted from our handheld devices and computer screens, light that turns off the production of melatonin and can completely disrupt our circadian rhythm.[10]

Technology can also lead to problems staying asleep, plus sleep deprivation. You may hear friends and family talk about their new blue-light blocking glasses and wonder if you should hop on the trend. In my opinion, it's a great and easy way to counteract the adverse effects of staring at a screen all day. There are also apps and software that can block blue light. Many phones have features in their display settings, as well, to reduce blue light or turn it off completely.

Adjusting your environment to counteract overstimulation and light exposure can make a difference. Each is a stress signal to your brain. If you have a lot of electronics in your bedroom, like speakers, charging stations, a clock, and a television, you'll probably notice that each of these items has its own light source. The best solution? Remove them from your bedroom. Or, at the very least, cover up the light they emit. You can buy stickers to black out the lights. You may not feel that a little ambient light here or there makes a difference, but it does. Any light that our brain perceives triggers a decrease in melatonin.

Our mobile devices act as many things: alarm clocks, newspapers, computers, televisions . . . the list goes on. But they can be a stress source. Similarly, having a TV in your bedroom can contribute to sleep deprivation. While TV in bed may feel like a luxury, it's probably a factor in your sleep problems. Not only do TVs emit blue light, but they also often turn into a temptation when you can't sleep. Many people find that removing the TV and even their phone from the bedroom can make a significant difference in sleep.

It's equally important to keep your blinds open during the day. Exposing yourself to natural light in the morning is crucial to helping your body establish and maintain a healthy circadian rhythm. This could mean meditating or exercising outside in the morning, going for a walk with your four-legged friends, or even moving your desk so that it is next to a window. In the winter, you may want to consider getting a light box to expose yourself to light in the morning to emphasize the circadian rhythm and give your body and brain the signals it needs to maintain your sleep-wake cycle. In fact, red light in particular is known to increase melatonin levels. Red-light therapy (known as photobiomodulation) has also been shown to reduce inflammation, oxidative stress, and other effects of stress, which means it can help you sleep well and feel better overall.[11]

I also recommend having a plant in your bedroom because plants are known to process toxins in the air and provide a view of nature for your brain. Your plant(s) will need sunlight during the day, just like you!

## Smell

Evidence shows that certain smells may have an effect on your sleep. That's because information about smells is sent to the limbic system and amygdala, via the olfactory nerve, connecting with emotions and memory. Aromatherapy is an ancient practice of using smells to relieve stress and anxiety and to improve mood and sleep.

For example, lavender essential oil has been shown to decrease stress levels and help with sleep.[12] There are several other essential oils known to promote relaxation, including vanilla, rose, geranium, and jasmine. You can add essential oils to your bath, use a diffuser, or simply use a spray bottle to mist your bed linens. Essential oils are concentrated, so don't apply them directly to your skin (and don't swallow them). It is best to dilute them in water for misting or in oil for applying to your skin. Adding a stress-reducing oil for your olfactory senses just might give you the extra encouragement you need to disconnect. If you have a pet, however, be aware that some essential oils are harmful to animals even if they are not in direct contact with the oils. It is best to research the oils you are thinking of using to be sure they are safe for your pets.

At the same time, when it comes to the air in your bedroom, it's also important to consider allergens and toxins. Especially if you have a tendency toward allergies to dust, mold, or pet dander, you'll want to choose hypoallergenic (and organic) bedding and mattress/pillow covers. Close your closet door or put your clothes inside drawers or containers. Clean regularly and get a high-quality air filter, with both HEPA and carbon filters, to filter out allergens as well as toxins. Toxins can enter your bedroom from car exhaust if you live on a busy road, or from your clothes if you use a dry cleaner. If at all possible, choose organic dry cleaning, and remove the plastic wrap from dry-cleaned clothes outside, before bringing them into your bedroom.

Be sure to also change the filter in your furnace and clean your air ducts on a regular basis. There are companies that use nontoxic, plant-based cleansers to clean air ducts. Keep an eye out for mold, which releases toxins into the air that get into your body and cause much more than sleep issues. Mold toxins, or mycotoxins, are among the most toxic compounds we come in contact with, and exposure happens more often than we'd think, because mold can grow where we don't see it: in crawl spaces, air ducts, air-conditioning units, and walls that have been water damaged.

## Sound

Sound is a key to sleep quality. Sounds can be both positive and negative influences on sleep. It depends on the type of sound you experience, the noise level, and your personal preferences and reactions to sound. Sounds that may seem trivial during the day often take their toll during the night. Consider environmental noise from road traffic, trains, planes, pets, phones, and city noise. So, how do you counteract this, especially if you live in areas with high noise pollution? For me, I love to throw on a sleep playlist from YouTube. If you're extremely sensitive to sound, consider including ear plugs as part of your bedtime routine. Also, be sure to put your smartphone on "do not disturb." There are settings that allow certain phone numbers to bypass "do not disturb," in case you don't want to miss a call from a loved one. There is also a setting that enables you to preset your bedtime and wake-up time, so that your phone automatically goes into "do not disturb" mode for the same hours each day.

On the other hand, certain types of sounds, like white noise, can moderate intermittent noise levels and act as a persistent backdrop for more peaceful rest. There's also pink noise. Both pink and white noise contain all the frequencies that are audible to humans. White noise has an equal amount of all the frequencies, but with pink, the lower frequencies are louder and have more power to reduce our brain waves, thus inducing sleep. Examples of pink noise in nature include raindrops, rustling leaves, and a heartbeat.

Every cell in our bodies is sensitive to frequency and vibration. Biochemists use sound waves with 528 Hz frequency to repair DNA. When we perceive a vibration that causes a sensation, like a tickle or tingle, it can cause relaxation and even help us to fall to sleep. This type of response is called autonomous sensory meridian response (ASMR). It can also be triggered by light touch or sound, and can feel like a shiver, telling you that your nervous system is calming down and shifting brain waves. ASMR has been associated with improved mood and decreased pain.[13] Pull up YouTube and search for music with 528

Hz or ASMR if you have trouble sleeping; maybe this will help you fall asleep or, at the very least, relax.

Some people are particularly sensitive to electromagnetic fields (EMFs) from Wi-Fi signals. Even though we can't hear them, our nervous system can pick up on these frequencies, which can disrupt sleep and adversely affect other areas of our health.[14] If that's the case for you, you may want to keep your cell phone out of your bedroom or turn it off; you can turn off the router in your home as well.

## Touch

One thing that will completely derail your sleep is feeling uncomfortable. If you're not sleeping well because you're waking up with aches and pains, it may be time for you to look into getting a new mattress. I recommend that you replace your mattress at least every ten years. Your pillows and their material should also suit your sleeping style. Perhaps you have joint hypermobility like me, so you may need to find the perfect pillows to support your neck and to prop up your knees a bit. Experiment and play around, but keep in mind that maintaining the most neutral position possible, with your neck supported, will help your body tremendously.

When you shop for a new mattress and pillows, choose organic ones. It absolutely makes a difference. Memory foam mattresses are filled with flame retardants, which can be absorbed by our bodies. This happened to me! Essentially, the very place I went to rest was affecting my body's ability to heal. I was always tired and in pain, and never felt like I fully recovered. It took me decades to discover that my body was filled with flame retardant, and ever since switching to an organic mattress, I've seen a significant difference. Luckily, today there are a lot of companies that offer high-quality organic mattresses and pillows. But they are not all created equal. It's worth your time to research and ask questions. Every part of the mattress, including the cotton, wool, and latex, should be organic. The top mattress brands I have found and use are Samina and Plushbeds. I've also switched to organic sheets and blankets from Coyuchi, but you can even find them at Garnet Hill, Anthropologie, or Target.

It's also important to consider the temperature of your room. Interestingly, we actually sleep better at a lower temperature: 60 to 67 degrees Fahrenheit. If it's too warm or cold in your room, it can be more difficult to fall asleep and/ or stay asleep. This is especially the case if you are experiencing night sweats due to hormonal shifts, such as during your menstrual cycle or menopause. Choosing the temperature in your bedroom is very personal, so you'll need to adjust to see what works best for you. There are also pads you can purchase to lie on that help keep you cooler while you sleep.

### Taste

Your palette comes into play in a variety of ways regarding your sleep hygiene. First and foremost, consider your diet. Yes, what you eat or drink during the day, plus any food sensitivities you might have, can positively or negatively affect your ability to snooze. In fact, not only what you eat, but when and how much you eat, affects your blood sugar levels, which in turn affects your sleep. If you find yourself waking up due to hunger in the middle of the night, you might need to examine your diet and how frequently you're taking time to eat during the day. Avoid carbs at night and keep meals light and protein-forward. Make sure you finish your last meal of the day at least two hours before you go to bed, and three hours would be better.

Additionally, food sensitivities such as to dairy and gluten, which cause inflammation and sinus congestion in certain people, can affect your ability to breathe while you sleep. This can show up in the form of heavy chronic snoring, sleep apnea, teeth grinding, and headaches. Leaky gut and imbalanced gut bacteria, associated with food sensitivities, can also disrupt sleep by increasing inflammation and weight gain and disrupting the nervous system via the gut-brain axis. If you are struggling with sleep, be sure to address your gut health.

## Sound Sleep Is Within Your Reach

It's easy to overlook the significance of sensory cues while you're asleep. But our environment, our daily routines, and our activities matter from dusk until dawn. Just because you think you've shut off your body and brain doesn't mean that you actually have. In fact, if you are like me and worry about your safety while you sleep, I encourage you to get a home alarm system and put an extra dead bolt on every door to prevent entry.

Once your sleeping space is all set, based on the sleep hygiene tips that we've discussed, all you need is a stress-reducing bedtime routine. I encourage you to start thinking about going to sleep at least an hour before you plan to fall asleep. Start by thinking of your dark, cozy, organic bedroom. Turn down the lights wherever you are and turn off your devices (or put on blue-light-blocking glasses) to decrease light exposure; this encourages your melatonin to increase. Drink herbal tea, such as chamomile, which is a calming herb, and take your last supplements at least an hour before bed so that you have time to pee before going to sleep.

Plan on meditating and/or taking a warm shower or bath (104 to 108 degrees Fahrenheit) for ten minutes before bed. This has been shown to improve sleep quality and quantity.[15] It can also increase slow-wave deep sleep by at least ten minutes early in the night.

In terms of eating, it's better to stay away from carbs close to bedtime, even though they tend to be what we crave most at night. In fact, a study showed that a high-carbohydrate, low-fat diet caused a decrease in slow-wave sleep. It's the oxidation of carbohydrates that suppresses slow-wave deep sleep. Studies are also starting to show that a fast-mimicking diet and intermittent fasting can increase deep sleep.[16] Your final meal should not be super high carb (as a classic dessert would be) and should not be too close to bedtime. Focus on eating protein and fats instead of carbs, and stop eating at least two hours before bed.

Even though many people turn to drinking alcohol in the evening to "relax" and "de-stress," studies show that alcohol is known to impair deep sleep. Caffeine and nicotine decrease deep sleep, as well.[17] So, as tempting as it is to have a piece of chocolate, which contains caffeine, and work on your computer at night, this is actually working against you because it detracts from deep sleep. Another important tip: while exercising too close to bedtime can inhibit sleep, especially for Night Owls, exercise in the evening has actually been shown to push REM sleep farther out into the night (early-morning hours), which increases deep sleep early in the evening.

To encourage tight muscles to relax, neck and shoulder muscles in particular, apply magnesium oil or lotion, and/or CBD and THC (cannabinoids, which I'll discuss further in chapter eight) topical oil or salve. Apply moisturizing lotion to your hands and feet—preferably organic, toxin-free, and gluten-free—which is a nice way to give a self-massage, release relaxing endorphins, and replenish your skin while you sleep. Another idea is to apply castor oil topically—I like to use a roll-on applicator to make it less messy—to tight muscles, sore joints, and areas that need more lymphatic drainage, such as the armpits, liver, and chest area. This makes for a pleasant bedtime ritual that can also help you fall asleep faster.

If you're not able to fall asleep after twenty minutes, do something that will calm your mind. Perhaps a light stretch, a meditation, or a progressive relaxation referred to as yoga nidra. Lie on your back, close your eyes, and breathe while bringing your attention to each part of your body, one by one, and then as a whole. Search online or on YouTube for a guided yoga nidra session, lasting between fifteen minutes and an hour. In fact, during meditation, brain waves can shift to alpha, theta, and even gamma waves, all of which provide beneficial rest for your brain. So, if you are not able to sleep, meditation is a smart alternative and may even help you fall asleep. Many people choose to read when they can't sleep, but reading requires light and, for some, may activate the brain, in which case it's better to read when not in bed.

Many people turn to sleep medications to help them get to sleep, which can be necessary for extreme cases and short periods of time. It is important to know that sleep medications are associated with worse cognitive function and they don't improve sleep characteristics (quality of sleep). Trazadone is the only medication shown to improve deep sleep; however, it is highly addictive and should be used only in extreme cases and under the supervision of a doctor.

If you are really struggling with sleep, and if you have been changing time zones or working the night shift, you may need to plan an opportunity to sync up your circadian rhythm. You could do this by going camping, an experience in which it gets dark when the sun goes down and you are exposed to the stars and moon while you sleep and the sunrise when you wake. You could also emphasize the spiritual elements of earth, fire, water, and air whether at home or at a retreat. Allow your senses to see, feel, or observe these aspects of nature—breathe fresh air, listen to the sound of a river, feel the warmth of a fire, and lie on the ground—all of which reset your stress response and body rhythms, including the sleep-wake cycle.

## Supplements for Sleep

As you implement Phase 1 of the Stress Recovery Protocol and work your way out of stress mode by dropping your elevated cortisol and adrenaline levels, you'll likely experience improved sleep.

Discovering whether you have low serotonin and/or GABA is also extremely helpful because then you can go through the process described in chapter ten in which you use precursor amino acids (5-HTP and theanine, respectively) to optimize your calming neurotransmitters, which you need in order to calm your brain for sleep. Balancing your blood sugar levels, addressing leaky gut, and optimizing your gut bacteria will also help with sleep over time.

If you need faster assistance to get more shut-eye, here are a few supplements to consider, all of which are nonaddictive.

Depending on where you live, melatonin may be available in products over the counter. Otherwise, it will require a prescription. Although it is preferable that our own bodies make melatonin for us, while you're adjusting your sleep routine and starting to implement C.A.R.E., it is okay to take melatonin. The common dosages are 1 to 10 mg, taken at about 10 PM or bedtime. Melatonin has also been shown to be effective for jet lag.[18] It is considered to be generally safe.

Valerian and other herbs that are calming, such as passionflower, lemon balm, chamomile, and California poppy, are all okay to try. You can get them as a tincture, in a capsule, or even as a tea. The dosing for these herbs is generally 200 to 500 mg each. They are considered safe, but I always caution people to look for any new or different symptoms, which could be caused by a reaction or allergy to an herb.

Magnesium is calming overall, decreases adrenaline, and relaxes muscle tension. Magnesium glycinate and threonate are the best options for these purposes, but if you have constipation and need help moving your bowels, you might choose magnesium citrate or oxide at bedtime to promote a bowel movement in the morning.

Glycine is an amino acid that is known to be calming to the nervous system and can help with sleep. It has been shown to improve sleep quality and promote deeper sleep. The dose is 3 to 5 grams before bed.

The classic homeopathic remedy for sleep is coffea cruda. Homeopathy is based on a system of dilutions and opposites. This means that coffee, which is stimulating in the usual amount, is calming in a homeopathic dilution. You can find homeopathic remedies over the counter. Look for the dose 30C and dissolve three pellets in your mouth before bed.

## Sleep for Your Stress Type

If you are struggling with sleep, there's a lot that you can do to help get your cycle back on track. Let's talk it through from the perspective of each stress type. Do keep in mind that it can take time for your body to adjust to new sleep and wake times. Studies show that even a difference of one hour, such as the change that happens with daylight saving time adjustments in the United States twice per year, leads to an increase in fatigue and car accidents for days after the change. Add in additional factors like travel and jet lag, and it can take weeks to readjust.[19]

A few years ago, I flew to Mumbai, India, from New York, which is about an eleven-hour time difference. I was there for two weeks to visit my sister and her family, who were living there at the time. When I flew home, it took me an entire month to get back on New York time and feel good. A month later, I flew to Manila, in the Philippines, to conduct presentations as a speaker and author on the topic of stress recovery. I was there for a week, and upon returning home, I once again needed a month to get my sleep pattern on track, even though I was using all the tools and techniques I've shared with you here. So please don't expect your body to adjust overnight. You can expect a shift of about thirty to sixty minutes each night.

One often-successful method of sleep recovery is to first narrow your window of sleep. If you're going to sleep and waking up after several hours, you may actually be going to sleep too early for your body. Start by staying up later and going to bed when you absolutely can't keep your eyes open anymore. Then, when you wake, stay up for the day. At first, you may get only four to six hours of sleep. From there, you can gradually add thirty to sixty minutes of sleep by going to bed earlier. Just remember to go slowly so your body has a chance to adjust, effectively retraining your circadian rhythm. I find that this technique is especially effective when people also address the issues specific to their stress types and follow my Stress Recovery Protocol.

## Stress Magnet

In your case, the most common scenario is waking up too early in the morning. This can be due to elevated cortisol alone or a combination of elevated cortisol and adrenaline that increases in the early hours. Think of this imbalance as your body trying to protect you from stress. It ends up waking you up, often with a rush of anxiety or a long list of things to do. Your heart may be racing, or you may get heart palpitations, and your mind just won't allow you to go back to sleep.

It's important to evaluate your neurotransmitter levels, such as serotonin and GABA, as well as your melatonin level, which can all be measured in a urine test from a specialty lab. Then follow my Stress Recovery Protocol to support your calming neurotransmitters using amino acid therapy: see chapter ten. Use magnesium threonate to decrease adrenaline that is too high. And use phosphatidylserine combined with herbs, such as banaba leaf or magnolia root, to calm down the cortisol production and reset the HPA axis. Depending on the severity of your sleep problems, you may need to take doses before you go to sleep, as well as when you wake up, and increase the doses until you are finding that you are sleeping longer (not waking up as early). Gradually, as you sleep later and your levels optimize, you won't need to continue taking these supplements unless the stress is unrelenting, in which case you can continue for as long as needed.

Stress recovery techniques, which we are going to discuss in detail in the next chapter, will also be helpful before you go to sleep and when you wake up. Meditation, for example, and really any form of mindfulness or relaxation technique, including deep breathing or biofeedback, can be helpful to counteract the stress signal to your brain. You'll essentially be retraining your nervous system to recognize that this is the time to relax and recover.

## Night Owl

Remember that your issue is that cortisol and adrenaline are increasing in the evening, instead of following a nice downward trend toward sleep. It's almost like you're living in the wrong time zone or your body thinks you're working the night shift. In fact, your body might literally lose track of day and night. This is simply an effect of stress.

You need to restructure your whole day. Yes, I'm putting the focus on daytime rather than nighttime. If you've been exercising for long hours, it may be time to take a break because a long run or training session can actually increase your cortisol level right up to when you're ready to sleep. Are you stressed at home, at work, or in your relationships? Was there a death in the family, a move, a divorce, a deadline? These are the types of stresses that can cause your body to lose track of your circadian rhythm. Are you skipping meals all day? Do you have digestive issues, joint pain, or other inflammation in your body that needs to be addressed? Your body is telling you it is time to address these problems, and not just with pain meds and antacids. You need to get to the root of the issue.

If your situation is severe, it's important to work with a practitioner who can guide you to do specialty tests for food sensitivities, imbalanced gut bacteria, mycotoxins, and genetic variations, in addition to cortisol and neurotransmitters, so that you have the information you need to create a strategic plan to recover. Getting your sleep back on track starts with balancing your blood sugar levels during the day by eating consistent meals that you can digest easily and that don't increase inflammation in your body. Stay hydrated throughout the day, and practice stress recovery activities. You essentially need to override the stress signal with anti-stress factors.

To begin, start by implementing C.A.R.E. as described in this book, as well as Phase 1 of the Stress Recovery Protocol. You'll want to match the timing of your doses of phosphatidylserine and banaba leaf (or another herb that decreases cortisol) with the times of day when your cortisol tends to increase. So, if your cortisol tends to start going up at 5 PM, take your dose at 4 PM. And if your cortisol continues to increase through the evening, take an additional dose every two to four hours until you go to sleep. Increase the dose until you find the amount that overrides the cortisol signal. To achieve this result, some people may need only one or two capsules of phosphatidylserine each night, within an hour or so of bedtime. Others may have to start dosing early in the day or evening and repeat the doses two or three times in order to shift the pattern.

Once you notice that your cortisol has shifted and you're feeling calmer in the evening and falling to sleep more easily, you can gradually decrease the doses to be sure the effect sticks. If you start having issues again, simply increase the doses again. If you find that you feel better, you can stop taking the phosphatidylserine and herbs to decrease cortisol and go back to them if needed in the future. Remember, it takes the body time to adjust your sleep-wake cycle.

## Sluggish and Stressed

While you may sleep just fine, having high cortisol in the morning, even without high adrenaline, can still cause you to wake up early. You may wake to a boost of energy that you welcome because it contrasts with how you feel the rest of the day. Or you may wake to a rush of stress and worry as soon as you open your eyes. Before long, as the cortisol awakening response completes and your cortisol levels begin to decrease or even drop, you may feel like you've run out of steam, especially because your adrenaline is also low. Be careful not to overdo caffeine, which could disrupt your ability to fall asleep at a good time in the evening.

Like the Stress Magnet, you may need to take a supplement at bedtime to prevent cortisol from rising so much in the early morning. That's the best way to get ahead of the cortisol before it has a chance to rise too high. You can also take a dose immediately upon waking, to continue to signal your body that you don't need so much cortisol in the morning. Gradually the HPA axis will reset, and you'll feel better in the morning—with energy but without such a rush of stress. That's when you'll be able to start supporting your adrenaline levels, so that you are getting energy from healthy adrenaline instead of from unhealthy cortisol.

Be sure to include stress recovery activities before you go to sleep, and plan on a meditation when you wake in the morning, to further signal to your body that you don't need so much cortisol to protect you.

## Blah and Blue

You may actually find that your issue with sleep is that you could sleep all day if your schedule allowed it. When cortisol doesn't increase in the morning, and neither does adrenaline, you never really get that "it's morning, and time to get up" feeling. The challenge is more about how to drag yourself out of bed without a million alarms going off. At the same time, if you, like some people in the Blah and Blue stress type, also find it hard to turn off your brain and body and go to sleep at night, you may actually be short on hours of sleep.

First, be sure you have enough serotonin and GABA, so get a neurotransmitter panel done and address them first. Even though you are exhausted after a night of rest, if you start boosting your cortisol and adrenaline without having enough serotonin and GABA, it will be like pressing on the gas pedal without having any brakes. Build up your brake system first, which will also help you get to sleep at an earlier bedtime and get more deep sleep. This way, when it's time to wake up, you will be more likely to have better energy.

Then, once you've got the calming system in place (in Phase 1 of the Stress Recovery Protocol), you can start supporting your cortisol and adrenaline in the morning and retraining your awakening response. You'll definitely benefit from walking through the sleep hygiene tips in this chapter and thinking about what you can do to make your bedroom a sanctuary. I say this because often my Blah and Blue patients have felt so exhausted and overwhelmed for so long that they are likely to have piles of laundry and clutter, and perhaps they haven't "had time" to order themselves new organic bedding and blackout shades. To which I say, "It's time to put you on the to-do list!"

Make a list and work through the tasks one by one. You don't have to get them all done in a day, but it will make a difference when your adrenals can get every ounce of recovery time while you sleep. That's the thing: all this time you've been in bed, but you haven't been getting the deep sleep your adrenals needed in order to recover.

## Tired and Wired

High adrenaline can cause you to feel revved up when trying to sleep. It can also cause you to wake in the middle of the night or early in the morning, with your heart racing and your body sweating. All of this can make you feel anxious. You might wonder if there's something wrong with your body or heart. Definitely check with your cardiologist. But it very well may be that adrenaline is kicking in even when you're not stressed.

Try taking magnesium threonate before bed and when you wake up. You can also add vitamin B6 to help COMT metabolize adrenaline more efficiently. You may have digestive issues to address, including overgrowing gut bacteria and leaky gut, which decrease the metabolism of adrenaline and work against you. You may also be drinking too much alcohol or exposing yourself to toxins that affect how your body processes adrenaline. Take all these factors into consideration, and then implement the sleep tips mentioned in this chapter to give your body the right signals for sleep, and not stress.

The stress recovery activities that we are going to talk about in chapter eight will be essential for you to integrate before you go to bed, if you wake in the middle of the night, and when you wake in the morning. You need lots of anti-stress tactics to reteach your body to turn on the parasympathetic nervous system. If and when you wake in the middle of the night, train yourself to go straight to turning on calming music, taking deep breaths, and reassuring yourself that sleep is in your future (instead of allowing the stress from not sleeping to make everything feel worse). This is also helpful when your sleep is cut short by other activities or travel. It's no use to stress about it. It's better to be proactive about giving your body rest in another form.

# *R* for Recovery

Recently, I was talking with a patient, Carol, and her soon-to-be second husband, Sean, about how stress related to their health issues. Carol, who is sixty-two years old, had abnormal cells on her cervix (caused by the HPV virus), and Sean had prostate cancer. They had both experienced severe stresses throughout their lives and had recently found love with each other. Now they wanted to be able to live without stressful drama and without the health issues caused by stress. They wanted to better understand both the effects of stress and, just as important, how to effectively recover from stress.

As Carol was busy taking notes, ordering products, and putting her supplement doses into her calendar, Sean laughed. He joked that she kept herself so busy every minute of every day. Now she was taking care of him, too. His tone then shifted toward worry: he didn't know when she'd have time for practicing stress recovery.

I pointed out that taking care of him was her way of showing her love and staying busy, which can be a stress recovery technique for some. And I emphasized to her that stress recovery activities are not the same as being lazy or doing nothing, although she admitted learning the opposite from her parents when she was a child.

Actually, a lot gets done when we are doing stress recovery. The parasympathetic and sympathetic nervous systems reset. The hypothalamus receives a signal to turn off the stress response. The digestive system gets the signal to digest and absorb nutrients. Those nutrients then go to our cells and tissue, where repair can happen, instead of going to fat storage and inflammation, where cell damage occurs. The mitochondria, brain, and liver clear out toxins. New neural pathways can form (the brain's ability to do this is referred to as neuroplasticity).[1] We can breathe in oxygen, process emotions, and find ourselves again, amid the chaos.

We've spent some time exploring how the messengers (hormones, neurotransmitters, and so on) inside our bodies get disrupted by stress for the different stress types. Choosing stress recovery activities is imperative, but so is addressing the imbalances caused by stress. When we do the stress recovery activities without addressing what was thrown off by stress, very little changes in the long term. Inevitably, our bodies revert to their stressed states. This is why it is important to combine my Stress Recovery Protocol (outlined in part three) with the stress recovery activities I'm about to share with you in this chapter in order to restore balance, little by little, and produce lasting changes.

## Using Self-Care to Your Benefit

Have you ever felt like you just want to sit on a beach and listen to the waves?

That's what Carol described as her perfect idea of a "day off."

Carol was correct—sitting on the beach listening to the waves is a beautiful way to reset from stress.

"How can you bring that same feeling and experience into your usual day?" I asked.

When she realized that adding stress recovery to her usual to-do list would feel overwhelming, I encouraged her to think about stress recovery as essential activities (in which she gets a lot of healing done inside her body) that are separate from her to-do list. I also think of stress recovery as self-care. We talked about how she could plan a time in the morning and the middle of the day when she could close her computer, turn on the sound of ocean waves, take some deep breaths, and imagine the waves washing her stress away.

So, what is self-care? Well, exactly what Carol was doing with those waves. However, for a long time, self-care was thought to be little more than indulgences and pampering, such as getting a massage, having a pedicure, or sitting on the couch eating bonbons. It was seen by some as choosing to "be lazy," and it had a significant stigma.

I get it. I grew up with that way of thinking, too.

Self-care, though, is an essential human need. It's not something to feel bad about or wait for your one week of vacation per year to practice. I once had a patient tell me she'd been waiting for her week of vacation to treat herself to self-care. On the first day of her vacation, her apartment flooded. She had to spend the whole week cleaning up the mess instead of relaxing. That's when she realized that it doesn't work to procrastinate stress recovery. Without regular self-care, we work against ourselves. And by judging ourselves for choosing self-care, we create more stress than we had to begin with!

Please don't feel that you have to do everything mentioned in this chapter to heal. Not everyone enjoys or benefits from the same self-care routine or stress recovery activities. And it's been proven that stressing about stress and self-care makes matters worse for a burned-out body. It's time to set aside any perfectionist tendencies and allow for curiosity and playfulness.

It's okay to start small. Don't downplay the positive effects of simple activities that help you recover from stress. When my daughter was young, having the chance to take a long, hot shower was a rare and cherished event! Showering is a meditation for me to this day.

Think of when you were a child. Recall your excitement to try new things, to learn and grow. Are there activities you enjoyed as a child but haven't tried for a long time? Those may be perfect stress recovery activities to consider bringing back now.

I was a dancer growing up and through college. I danced in competitions and on football fields. I taught dance in college and to children as a part-time job when I was in medical school. Then, after becoming a doctor, I stopped dancing. I drove my daughter to many dance classes, but never danced myself, until two years ago. I signed up for ballroom dance classes. It was one of the best things I've ever done in terms of self-care and stress recovery. Within six months, I was performing again and loving every minute of it.

It's also okay to start with what you already do. When someone asks you what your hobby is, are you the person who doesn't have a reply? I was that person. For a long time, my hobby was cooking and cleaning, because that's what I did the most (and what I had to do). I find that reframing what you do as part of your stress reduction can allow you to see it in a new light. Washing the dishes can be a great way to practice mindfulness. Reading stories to your children allows you to practice being present in the moment. Walking your dog helps you as much as it does your dog. So do watering the plants and drinking a cup of tea. The key is to do these activities with a mindset of stress recovery.

Another way to bring mindfulness to your self-care is to integrate the elements of nature discussed in chapter five—earth, fire, water, and air. By associating significance with your choices, you bring spirituality into your daily existence. For example, you can choose activities that allow you to focus on and enjoy the four elements. Going to the beach, taking a hike, and even sitting on the grass are all ways to connect with earth. Build a fire in the fireplace, or light a toxin-free, natural candle or incense to experience fire. Drink filtered water or herbal tea with intention and take a shower or bath, or even a swim in a lake or the ocean, to connect with water. Practice breathing techniques, or whistle or sing, to be present with air.

## Draw a Boundary That Works for You

Often the hardest part about choosing stress recovery activities is that it means you'll need to say no to someone or something else to create the time and space for stress reduction.

It's also possible that others in your life may want to join you. In fact, connection with others is a great self-care activity. If codependency is an issue for you, choosing self-care can feel difficult at first. If you notice that you feel anxious or guilty for choosing to take care of yourself, take a deep breath and just pay attention to the feeling. This is part of stress reduction—just being present and gaining confidence in feeling your feelings. You deserve to take care of yourself and feel good.

Choose to allow *what you want* to be more important than what others want at this moment. You can choose it gently while also setting a boundary: that this is your time, for you.

Let's look at practices you can choose for your stress recovery time.

## Be Grateful

Let's start with gratitude.

Being in a state of gratitude reduces stress, as well as cortisol and blood pressure that are too high—all while improving sleep and mood. Feeling grateful even for a few minutes can create a long-lasting feeling of happiness by increasing serotonin and dopamine levels and works whether you communicate your gratefulness to another person or not. When we feel appreciation on a regular basis, we become more resilient to setbacks and are able to recover from stress faster.[2] And what's more, when we consistently practice gratitude, the brain gets better at choosing and experiencing gratitude.[3]

Gratitude is also known to increase oxytocin.[4] Once thought to be associated only with birth and breastfeeding (as a bonding hormone), now we know that men also make oxytocin and that it acts as a stress recovery hormone. It is produced when we are stressed to help us cope with danger. Oxytocin decreases anxiety, cortisol, and pain; and is an antioxidant and anti-inflammatory.[5] Our pituitary gland (in the brain) produces a background level of oxytocin all the time at a set point that seems to be determined by our genetics and past stress exposure. Then, when a stress comes along, the levels increase temporarily. Oxytocin is also produced by the heart and causes us to feel love and attraction (isn't that amazing?!).[6] You can give yourself a boost of this stress recovery hormone whenever you'd like, simply by choosing stress recovery activities such as gratitude.

To practice gratitude, start by taking a couple of deep breaths. Think of something or someone you feel grateful for right now. You might feel grateful for the place you are sitting, the people and pets in your life, for being alive, for something that happened today, for the food you ate, or for the air you breathe. It may help to say out loud or in your mind, "I'm thankful for . . ." Or you may want to write down what you feel grateful for in a gratitude journal (in other words, a journal that you solely devote to thankfulness).

Practice doing this each day, whether it's when you wake in the morning or before you go to sleep at night. It's amazing to me that even on the most stress-filled day, jammed with tasks to complete and issues to resolve, I can always think of something I'm grateful for. In doing so, I immediately feel a sense of relief. I feel that it's all going to be okay.

## The Power of Quiet

Sitting in silence is another example of how doing nothing, quite literally, can positively affect your brain and body. With two hours of silence in a day, a study showed growth of new hippocampus cells, which are important for memory, emotion, and learning.[7]

Now, if you are a parent, work, own your business, or have others to care for, it may be hard to imagine having two minutes—let alone two hours—of silence. Start with two minutes, and gradually find ways to increase this window. Can you block out fifteen minutes in your schedule? Can you set aside an hour on the weekend when you might usually do laundry and cleaning, or watch TV? What happens if you choose silence instead?

At first, you may feel like something is missing or like you are missing out on being somewhere. But once you allow yourself moments of silence, I think you'll see how valuable they are, and they will become easier to choose and even prioritize.

## Meditation

Take silence to another level by making it meditation.

Meditation is a state of being in the present moment. Many people think they are supposed to stop thinking to meditate, so it feels impossible. But actually, in meditation, thoughts still happen. It's just that you become better at noticing each thought and letting it go, without feeling that you need to do something or figure it out right now.

In fact, it's the opposite of concentrating and ruminating on thoughts. Meditation is about allowing your thoughts to be like sounds or breaths: they happen, but they don't have to cause you to respond. They come. You notice them. They pass. It's about being in the present, instead of thinking of the past or wondering about the future. And meditation is a practice, meaning there's no expectation or judgment about whether you are doing it correctly. It's a stress-free activity.

I learned how to meditate when I was in naturopathic medical school, at Bastyr University in Seattle, Washington. Meditation was a common activity, as were ceremonies and honoring one other and the medicine we were learning. I practiced meditation in various ways over the years—during yoga classes, at home, and at conferences. At a young age, my daughter noticed the cat sitting with her paws tucked under her chest and announced, "The cat is 'meowitating'!" Still, it wasn't until recently, when I attended a weeklong meditation retreat where I meditated for eight hours a day and learned advanced techniques, that I finally really experienced the full potential of meditation.

In a meditative state, you are relaxed but awake. You allow yourself to become no one, nowhere, doing nothing. By adding breath work, it's possible to reach states of deep relaxation and insight where you feel gratitude and self-love, which is a form of healing in itself. Physiologically, during meditation, brain waves shift from beta to alpha, theta, and/or gamma. The increase in theta waves indicates deep relaxation in the frontal and middle part of the brain, where mental processes occur. In the posterior (rear) area of the brain, alpha waves increase, indicating wakeful rest and a break from intentional tasks.[8] Delta waves, associated with sleep, and beta waves, associated with focusing on a task, are not predominant during mediation.

In people who meditate regularly, over time, they experience improved focus and decreased emotional reactivity to stress, indicating that neuroplasticity occurs with meditation.[9]

## Mindfulness

Mindfulness is a slight variation on meditation. It is simply the act of being present in the moment, whatever you are doing. A common place to start is by practicing mindful eating, as we talked about in chapter six.

A few years ago, I took a course called Mindfulness-Based Stress Reduction (MBSR), a well-researched program developed by the author Jon Kabat-Zinn. In the class, we learned a bunch of different ways to practice mindfulness. Everything from sitting or lying quietly to eating, walking, moving, stretching, writing, or talking mindfully. The class was held in the fall in a rustic building on a huge property that is essentially a park. Just being allowed to take a couple of hours each week to sit in that natural and beautiful environment with a group of people who all wanted to reduce stress and increase mindfulness was a life-changing experience.

Interestingly, several studies have shown that both meditation and mindfulness help whether your cortisol is too high or low. In cases where salivary or plasma (blood) cortisol was too high, meditation helped lower it to a more optimal level. And in cases where cortisol was too low, meditation increased cortisol to a more optimal level. That means meditation (and other forms of mindfulness) helps with all stress types. People who needed it most, and were most symptomatic, improved the most from an eight-week program, and the benefits seem to be maintained over time.[10]

## The Power of Spiritual Practice

In many ways, gratefulness, silence, meditation, and mindfulness are very similar to the experience of prayer. They are also all parts of different religious practices. The difference is that prayer often involves thought and communication directed to a god figure or object of worship, as a form of devotion, praise, and asking for help. Spirituality in general helps people feel connected to others and the world, which allows them to feel less like they need to control it all themselves. Feeling part of a greater whole makes it easier for them to understand that they are not responsible for everything that happens.

Studies have shown that prayer can help people cope with stress, as well. People who participate in prayer and religious services are less likely to need to visit the doctor's office, are less likely to experience depression, are less stressed even during difficult times, and have increased odds of living longer—all by 29 percent. Studies have also shown that such people are less likely to have a stroke, are less likely to die after heart surgery, and have shorter hospital stays than those who do not have a spiritual practice. Faith provides hope, which is more powerful than the placebo effect.[11]

You can also bring spirituality into your self-care time using the four elements discussed in chapter five: earth, fire, water, and air. You can do this by feeling gratitude for each of these elements in nature and what they make possible. By bringing our attention to the world around us, and ultimately the universe, it shifts our focus away from our daily stresses and helps us to see that we are part of a bigger whole.

## Biofeedback

Biofeedback is a technique involving breath and positive intentions to shift the response to stress, while also measuring a change in the body, such as a change in the heart rate. Interestingly, there is a pattern to our heart rate where it speeds up as we inhale and slows down as we exhale (referred to as respiratory sinus arrhythmia). The variation in the pattern, called heart rate variability (HRV), reflects our state of stress based on how stress affects the autonomic nervous system. When we feel negative or unpleasant emotions—such as anger, frustration, guilt, shame, and sadness—our heart rate becomes less variable (I know that seems opposite, but it is correct), or less coherent. In contrast, when we feel calmness, happiness, and love, our heart rate is more coherent and has more variance between heartbeats. A high HRV indicates better recovery from stress.[12]

We can increase our heart coherence by breathing in a ten-second rhythm (five seconds to breathe in and five seconds to breathe out), which in turn sends a signal of calmness to the brain and the rest of the body via the vagus nerve and parasympathetic nervous system. This is the mechanism used with biofeedback methods, such as a well-established method known as Heart-Math, of which I am a certified practitioner. Heart rate variability (HRV) is measured and monitored alongside the biofeedback techniques to help assess and demonstrate improvements in resiliency to stress and what is referred to as "vagal tone."[13]

You can learn, practice, and apply biofeedback techniques in real life to change how you respond to stress and help your body shift to the parasympathetic nervous system. This has been shown to improve memory, focus, and performance. These techniques increase alpha waves in the brain, the same waves associated with meditation. Biofeedback can be used by children, students, athletes, parents, and professionals, at any point in time, in the moment and as a way to shift their overall state. With biofeedback, you can choose in the moment to take steps to help with stress recovery and improve resilience to stress. Studies show a decrease in cortisol levels with biofeedback, as well as decreased muscle tension, and for those with high blood pressure, it brings blood pressure closer to normal (when blood pressure is normal, it stays normal).[14]

## Breath Work and Yoga

There are many ways you can improve HRV and vagal tone including breath work, such as heart-focused breathing, which involves a ten-second breathing pattern described above while also focusing on your heart area (it can help to put your hand over your heart). Then think of something or someone you love—a person or pet—or simply feel gratitude for a person or experience. You might do this first for one minute. Then you might lengthen the amount of time from five to fifteen minutes per day to help get yourself out of stress mode. By breathing this way, you'll become more able to respond in the stressful moments of your life, without feeling overwhelmed by the stress.

Yoga is an example of moving mindfully and is a form of spirituality; it can include chanting and singing and often ends with meditation. Yoga has been practiced for thousands of years and continues to be a popular way to de-stress and exercise. Studies show that cortisol levels do decrease after yoga.[15] It involves breath work, stretching, and poses, often in a series or progression, with the intention of reducing stress and negative thinking. There are several forms of yoga, including Kundalini, Vinyasa, Bikram (also known as hot yoga), Hatha, and Iyengar. It is important to choose a type of yoga that works well for you and your body. The whole idea behind yoga is for it to be non-harming, so it is not the place to push beyond your ability. Yoga is perfect when you want to feel connected with your body, something we lack in our busy lives.

## Animal Interactions

Spending time with animals is one of my favorite stress recovery activities. Perhaps some of you feel the same. Pets can provide enjoyment, connection, and snuggles. Whether you have cats, dogs, birds, horses, pigs, snakes, rabbits, ferrets, or any other animal in your home or on your property, I think you'll agree. While it does take time and effort to care for them, the benefits of having animals in your life are endless. Studies show that having a dog decreases heart disease risk, likely by providing social support and motivation to exercise. Having a cat can decrease risk of a stroke or heart attack by one-third.[16] This is likely because, as studies have shown, when people have a pet, they experience lower cortisol, adrenaline, stress and anxiety, and both blood pressure and heart rate decrease while HRV increases. Oxytocin is released when we bond with a pet, particularly when we pet (stroke) them, and is likely why we experience so many benefits.[17]

Please be mindful that when you take on a pet, it's your responsibility as a human to feed and take care of it. Because I run a feral cat rescue and care facility, I'm all too familiar with the inhumane treatment that can occur. If you allow your cat (or dog) to go outside, and especially without first having it fixed (spayed or neutered), you risk contributing to the huge population of cats that don't have a home. It is wonderful to adopt a pet, but abandoning it is neglectful. There are pet rescues in most towns that offer services for if you are no longer able to care for your pet. Please join me in caring for the animals that can provide such amazing stress reduction for us humans, when these animals have a loving home.

## Time in Nature

Spending time in nature is another great stress reducer.

Perhaps it comes from growing up in the Pacific Northwest of the United States, where there are so many outdoor activities, including hiking, skiing, and boating, but I find that even ten to fifteen minutes in nature can make a difference in my day.

One study found that cortisol decreases at a rate of 18 percent per hour even within the first twenty to thirty minutes of spending time in a natural, outdoor space.[18] Other studies have indicated that phytoncides, the aromatic volatile substances released by plants, can decrease adrenaline levels and increase natural killer (NK) cells, the part of our immune system that protects us from infections and tumors.[19]

*Shinrin-yoku*, which means "forest bathing," is a form of mindfulness in Japan and Asian countries that involves immersing oneself in nature. Studies have shown its benefits throughout the body, including the immune system, heart and lungs, and mind; it's also known to decrease anxiety and improve focus.[20]

The beneficial effect of nature is in part due to the negative ions in the air, which come from the ultraviolet (UV) rays of the sun, from plants, and from water that is colliding, such as a waterfall or waves hitting the shore. Studies have also demonstrated the benefits of being in contact with the earth; this is called electrically conductive contact and is also known as grounding or earthing. The earth is electromagnetic and gives off electrons. Our bodies also have electromagnetic fields in every cell and organ, which make it possible for them to function, move fluid and electrolytes, contract muscles, counteract oxidative stress, and essentially perform every activity in our bodies. Nerves in our bodies, including the vagus nerve we spoke about earlier in this chapter, all work by sending electrical signals. As we support the electrical signals through the vagus nerve, vagal tone improves and our bodies recover from stress.[21]

Let's think this through in a bit more detail. The vagus nerve is the main part of the parasympathetic nervous system (the anti-stress system) and a major part of communication between the gut and the brain (the gut-brain axis).[22] It also signals something called the "inflammatory reflex," which turns on inflammation when we have an injury or infection. When we are under chronic stress, vagal tone decreases, and inflammation increases, leading to autoimmunity and metabolic issues associated with obesity.[23]

When we are inside buildings and wearing shoes outdoors, we do not receive electrons from earth, leaving us vulnerable to inflammation. On the other hand, when we stand or walk barefoot on the ground, grass, or beach, free electrons spread into our bodies, acting as antioxidants and decreasing inflammation.[24] There are also grounding devices we can get for our homes and offices. As a related point, it is essential that we consume adequate electrolytes—sodium, potassium, calcium, and other trace minerals—to allow electrical signals to move through our bodies efficiently.

While I encourage you to find ways to spend time outside in nature whenever this is possible (and safe), I also like to emphasize ways to experience nature from indoors. Particularly if you are not able to go outdoors, for any reason, you can bring nature into your life by having a plant, looking at pictures of nature, or looking out the window. Gaze at the sky, sunset, sunrise, moon, fresh flowers, trees, birds, insects, snow, lake, or ocean. There is something about the colors and symmetry found in nature that our brain picks up on immediately. Studies of nature therapy show that the autonomic nervous system shifts into parasympathetic mode, heart rate variability improves, and cortisol stabilizes.[25] It's like we are preprogrammed to enjoy nature. You don't even have to try. Just sit and look, and your brain will take it from there.

## Hands, Meet Dirt. Dirt, Meet Hands.

Gardening is a perfect way to spend time in nature and has been studied in comparison to reading a book. Both activities resulted in a decrease in cortisol levels, but with gardening, the change was more significant.[26] Plus, with gardening, there was an improvement in mood that didn't occur with reading (I'm hoping this book *does* improve your mood!).

As with most activities, it's important to be mindful when gardening. Wear shoes or boots to protect your feet (unless you take them off for grounding!), and a hat, gloves, long sleeves, and pants to prevent ticks and other insects from biting you, and to prevent sunburn. Use kneepads when kneeling for long periods of time and essential oils, such as cedar, eucalyptus, and citronella, to fend off mosquitoes. You could also plant a few herbs (I like to plant basil, rosemary, and sage) or houseplants. Caring for them helps with stress, too.

## Laugh!

Often, we hear that laughter is one of the best medicines, and it's true! Studies show that watching a funny show and laughing out loud can reduce stress, and more specifically reduce cortisol and adrenaline.[27] Laughter has also been shown to improve circulation, decrease heart rate and blood pressure, decrease pain, and improve mood and immunity. That's because laughter boosts serotonin, a calming neurotransmitter, and causes a release of oxytocin, which helps us feel connected to others, and endorphins, which bind to opiate receptors relieving pain.[28]

Find ways to bring laughter into your life, perhaps by reading a funny book, watching a cartoon, or talking with friends who can make you laugh. My dog makes me laugh at all the funny things she does. Learning to laugh at ourselves tends to happen when we let go of our stresses. Let it happen; it's good for you!

## The Power of Sound and Movement

Music is another self-care tool that helps us recover from stress. Simply turning on tunes can melt away the day's stress. Studies show a decrease in cortisol and an increase in oxytocin after listening to music, and this is true for both slow-tempo and fast-tempo music.[29]

Music therapy is the use of music by a music therapist for healing. Music is used to help people express themselves, facilitate movement, and provide emotional support. Music medicine, on the other hand, is the use of music without a therapist. Studies have demonstrated improvements in mood, memory, and immunity from both music therapy and music medicine.[30] After spending time in Peru and in shaman ceremonies, I especially enjoy listening to *icaros*, which are the healing songs sung, whistled, or played on an instrument by a shaman, such as during an ayahuasca journey (I'll discuss in more detail shortly).

Sound therapy is the use of sound for healing and it is based on the concept that certain frequencies in sound can influence the frequencies inside our bodies (and brains), and help bring them to a level associated with health. The most healing frequencies (or tones), such as 528 and 432 Hz, were identified mathematically and were named Solfeggio frequencies (tones of a scale). They have been shown to decrease heart rate and stress more than other frequencies.[31] Binaural beat therapy uses sounds entering the left and right ears at slightly different frequencies. Proponents find that it reduces stress and anxiety and that it increases focus and motivation.[32] Safe and Sound Protocol (SSP) uses calming music to create a sense of safety via the vagus nerve.[33]

When we think about it, sound has been used for healing back in history and across cultures—for example, Himalayan singing bowls and Sanskrit chants. So turn up the tunes! And while you're at it, sing and dance to the music. Move. Vocalize. Recover.

Do you sing in the shower or while driving? If not, you might try it. Singing, humming, and chanting all stimulate the vagus nerve, helping to shift you into a parasympathetic state.[34] Or turn on some music and have a dance party break, by yourself or with your kids. There is a reason cultures around the world include music, singing, and dance as part of their celebrations. Some forms of dance can actually raise your cortisol and adrenaline, especially if the music is loud; this is also the case with drumming, which can be great exercise.[35]

I have fallen in love with ballroom dancing as both a form of exercise and a break from the stress of the day. Studies have shown that whether you are doing the foxtrot or line dancing, it has a positive effect on your brain, improving serotonin levels and making neural connections that stave off forms of dementia.[36]

## Sauna Therapy

In studies, a twenty-minute sauna twice a week resulted in an initial increase in norepinephrine and cortisol, which then decreased over time. Heat from the sauna relaxes muscles, improves circulation, and causes sweating, a well-established form of detoxification. At the same time, endorphins are released, which are feel-good, pain-relieving hormones. Infrared saunas provide heat from varying wavelengths, which benefits our bodies in different ways, from tissue healing and decreased inflammation to detoxification. Regular sauna use has been associated with decreased blood pressure, anxiety, and dementia.[37] Be sure to stay hydrated—drink water with electrolytes—before and after your sauna, and shower off at the end to prevent toxins from being reabsorbed through your skin.

## Sex

Sex is also a stress recovery activity. This includes experiencing pleasant sexual feelings with yourself. It's absolutely imperative that any sexual activity is done only with the consent of the other person. So please don't read this to mean that you ought to find someone to have sex with just to reduce your stress, because you would be increasing the other person's stress, and that is not the point. The goal is consensual sexual activity, enjoyed between two adults (or by yourself), which has been shown to reduce stress and improve mood and oxytocin levels.[38] By the way, more frequent hugs from your partner also increases oxytocin and lowers blood pressure.[39]

In relationships in which people had sex at least once per week, they experienced an increased sense of well-being and enjoyment of life, likely related to the increase in oxytocin that occurs with intimacy.[40] One study found that sexual activity twice per week decreased cardiovascular risk by 45 percent (whereas having sex less than once per month increases risk).[41] Another study showed having a higher frequency of orgasms decreased the death rate by 50 percent over a ten-year period.[42] Sexual activity is also associated with improved cognitive abilities in older adults.[43] If there are health issues preventing you from being sexually active, know that there are ways to help you resolve these issues, and it's worth it for your health and well-being.

## Reaching Out

Talking with a friend or therapist can make all the difference in the world. Calling your mom has also been studied as a form of stress reduction, especially for daughters.[44]

Expressing how we feel and feeling heard are so powerful for us as humans. These forms of communication lower cortisol and adrenaline while increasing serotonin and oxytocin. We then feel connection, compassion, and increased confidence in ourselves, including in our ability to feel different feelings. Journaling, or writing about your feelings, is also beneficial.[45]

When you think about it, we spend a lot of our lives avoiding unpleasant feelings, such as sadness, shame, vulnerability, embarrassment, guilt, and anger. We go to great lengths to avoid conversations and situations that may involve these feelings. Yet when we choose to feel these feelings, and express them, in a well-meaning way, they can shift our experience and life. My friend Dr. Joan Rosenberg, who is a psychologist, has studied this effect over her thirty-year career and writes about how feeling your feelings can improve your life.[46]

Many forms of psychotherapy, such as cognitive behavioral therapy (CBT), are based on the idea of talking with a trained therapist who can validate your experience and help you process the emotional stresses in your life.[47] Eye movement desensitization and reprocessing (EMDR) is a form of therapy that involves methods of distracting the conscious mind to allow for greater resolution of subconscious traumas. Studies have shown it to be particularly helpful for post-traumatic stress disorder (PTSD) and other types of panic disorders.[48] There are also neurofeedback therapy, the NeuroAffective Relational Model (NARM), somatic therapy, and clinical hypnotherapy, all of which have helped people recover from stressful experiences and resolve anxiety, depression, and other effects of stress. If you haven't already worked with a therapist or psychoanalyst, I encourage you to add this to your self-care plan.

And if you've tried therapy but you'd like additional support to understand yourself and your experiences, you may find it helpful to work with an expert with a different perspective and approach. Naturopathic doctors are trained in counseling, so they can be a good resource, and some have completed additional training. For example, I completed certification as a life coach using the Holistic Breakthrough Method, which is a process to guide you to let go of past traumas and conditioned ways of being so that you can be your authentic, loving self.

## Solitude

Another benefit in many of these stress recovery activities is that they give you alone time. Many of us live with, work with, and interact with other people much of the day, and are exposed to constant demands and stimulation. If your children are like my daughter, they likely have a radar that alerts them as soon as you're focused on a task, because that's exactly when they will ask you to help them with something. It can be hard to find a minute to spend by myself or a space in my home to spend it. This is so much the case that it can feel odd to finally have space and time alone.

Meanwhile, studies show that when we have solitude, we are able to discover new ways of knowing ourselves, interconnections in life, and our purpose, which is an antidote to stress, loneliness, and depression.[49] I encourage you to create alone time, and when you have it, even for one minute, choose one of the stress recovery activities in this chapter to try. Before you know it, you'll cherish time alone and help others have it, too.

## Stress Recovery from Nature

In addition to the nutrients and herbs used in the Stress Recovery Protocol to rebalance cortisol, adrenaline, and neurotransmitters (which will be covered in part three), there are many substances that are specifically used to help with stress recovery. I'm going to review a few of them here, namely cannabinoids, psychedelics, peptides, and herbs that support telomere length.

### Cannabinoids

We've talked about the nervous system, the digestive system, the immune system, and even the endocrine system (which makes hormones), but we have yet to talk about the endocannabinoid system (ECS). Recently discovered as a whole separate system within the human body, the ECS is composed of the receptors and enzymes involved in the production and signaling of cannabinoids produced within the human body. The two known endocannabinoids, anandamide and 2-AG (short for 2-arachidonoylglycerol), are synthesized on demand from fatlike molecules in cell membranes. They then bind to receptors throughout the body, including in the brain, helping to bring the body back to homeostasis.[50]

Think of the story of Goldilocks. She didn't want things too big or too small, too hot or too cold. She wanted them "just right." That's what our bodies want and need, too, in order to function optimally. But stress pushes our bodies away from this perfect middle ground. That's where endocannabinoids come in, to help shift us and our cellular function back to optimal. In this way, they help with stress recovery. Enzymes break down the endocannabinoids once their job is done.

Endocannabinoids have been shown to decrease inflammation in the body by communicating with the immune system. They also decrease pain and stress. This is also true of cannabinoids from cannabis and hemp plants, of which over eighty have been identified, including both tetrahydrocannabinol (THC) and cannabidiol (CBD). It is important to know that the reduction in stress from THC is dose dependent—low doses decrease stress, while high doses can increase anxiety.[51] THC (from cannabis) decreases adrenaline, but increases cortisol, which means it may help the Tired and Wired stress type but not Sluggish and Stressed.[52]

There are many strains or types of cannabis; some are more calming or sedative (indica) and others are not as calming (sativa). The whole flower can be smoked and inhaled, or ingested, or the oil can be extracted and formulated into liquids, capsules, or lotions that are applied topically. Be sure to check the legality of cannabis in your area—the law may require you to become certified to use cannabis for medical purposes. Other sources of cannabinoids include plants we consume frequently, such as broccoli, black pepper, carrots, echinacea, ginseng, cloves, cacao (which is used to make chocolate), and tea (black and green).

## Psychedelics

Cannabinoids, which are psychedelics, are known to help with anxiety and depression, as are other psychedelics, such as ketamine, MDMA (methylenedioxymethamphetamine, also known as ecstasy), psilocybin (from medicinal mushrooms), and ayahuasca.[53] They are entheogens, which are psychoactive substances, usually from a plant, that cause an altered state of consciousness with visions and spiritual insights. Although psychedelics were outlawed in the United States in the 1960s, recent research and clinical use has raised awareness for their effectiveness in helping with stress recovery, from PTSD in particular.[54] Through guided experiences, patients have been able to gain a greater awareness of themselves, attain an increased sense of connection with others, and decrease their anxiety and stress.[55] Psychedelics are also used to help with addictions and trauma-related disorders. They have been shown to help those who are facing death from cancer, perhaps one of the greatest experiences of stress imaginable.[56]

Some states and countries have legalized these substances and are beginning to provide access to them for stress recovery and establish protocols for their use. Based on my research and experience, I feel they are an important option to consider for stress recovery, depending on a person's situation and comfort level.

Ayahuasca in particular has shown positive results for mood and stress recovery.[57] Ayahuasca is a blend of two plants: the ayahuasca vine and the leaves from the chacruna shrub. The vines and leaves are brewed together for days, and the final product, which is a thick, black liquid, contains dimethyltryptamine (DMT) as well as the alkaloids in ayahuasca, including harmine and harmaline. The first time I took ayahuasca (in Peru, where it is legal) I said to myself, "This is the missing medicine for our nervous system and stress recovery." Through a gentle process, over two to three hours, I felt the ayahuasca (which translates to "rope of death") release any and all stress in my body and nervous system. It was a total vagus nerve reset and a release of everything that no longer served me (the death of what we no longer need, as the shaman explained). If you are considering the use of an entheogen, such as ayahuasca, be sure to consult with a practitioner trained in the use of psychedelics or an experienced shaman who can help you use it safely and effectively.

## Peptide Therapy

Peptides, as researched by Dr. Vladimir Khavinson in St. Petersburg, Russia, are substances made in the human body, and in animals, that have the ability to reset genetic expression after stress exposure. Dr. Khavinson studied peptides during the Cold War in an effort to help soldiers recover from the stress of battle. Not only were the peptides able to restore healthy function, but they also actually worked at a genetic level to undo the effects of stress, thereby having an "antiaging" effect. Dr. Khavinson has since discovered peptides for various tissues in the body, from the pineal gland to the bones, and everything in between. Peptide therapy is either animal derived or synthetic and is considered safe and effective; it can be taken orally, injected, or inhaled.[58]

I had the pleasure of meeting Dr. Khavinson in person in his clinic in St. Petersburg, the Institute of Bioregulation and Gerontology. He described his research over the past fifty years with great enthusiasm, explaining that the use of peptides has been shown to increase life span by 20 to 40 percent. During the course of his work, Dr. Khavinson has published over eight hundred scientific papers and received numerous awards, and he holds patents for the peptides he developed in Russia. The two peptides that he considers to be essential are pineal (related to hormone production) and thymus (related to immune system regulation). These are used in combination with peptides specific to the area of the body that is showing a need for support in recovering from stress.

## Support Telomere Length

Another treatment modality based on helping our genes recover from stress exposure is the use of diet, herbs, and stress reduction to restore telomere length. Telomeres are at the ends of our genes and act as a protection from stress, like the plastic at the end of a shoelace. However, as we are exposed to stress or oxidative stress, the telomeres shorten, leaving us vulnerable to damage in our genes. Additionally, each time the DNA is replicated, which happens all day long, the telomeres become shorter. As they do, the risk of damaging DNA that codes for important proteins increases.

Shortening of telomeres is what causes aging; therefore, telomere length is known to be associated with increased longevity. This means that by taking steps to recover from stress, we can improve telomere length, protect our DNA, and prevent health issues. There are tests now available, which you can order online and do at home, to determine your current telomere length and your relative age (based on the length of your telomeres). Then, as you implement the protocols in this book, you can retest as a way of monitoring your progress.

As you might imagine, once telomeres were discovered, researchers started looking for substances that could reverse the shortening of telomeres.

One way to do that is by increasing the activity of an enzyme called telomerase that maintains the length of telomeres. Of the substances discovered to increase telomerase activity, several of them are herbs, which interestingly are also herbs that have been used for thousands of years to prevent aging. One of these is astragalus, an antioxidant herb that is also known to support immune function, prevent cancer, decrease inflammation, and help balance sugar. Another is elderberry or sambucus, which is often used to support the immune system and help fend off viruses. Green tea, ginkgo, and milk thistle have also been shown to increase telomerase activity, in addition to their other beneficial effects.[59] There are products now available that contain a combination of these herbs for efficient access to telomere restoration.

It is important to note that telomerase activity is also increased by eating a healthy diet (that is, by following the suggestions in chapter six); by participating in the stress recovery activities covered in this chapter, especially meditation; and by exercising (which we'll discuss in chapter nine). That means that one of the ways C.A.R.E. helps you recover and become resilient to stress is by helping to prevent damage to your telomeres.

There are many other substances and practices known to help the body shift out of stress mode, including homeopathic remedies, essential oils, and energy and touch therapies like Emotional Freedom Technique (EFT), Reiki, massage, and acupuncture.[60] Even a ten-minute massage or treatment can increase HRV indicating the vagus nerve has shifted to a parasympathetic state, helping you to reset your stress response.[61]

On the one hand, it is mind-blowing to think that we are surrounded on Earth with substances from nature and activities in nature or by human touch that help us heal and recover from stress. On the other hand, it makes sense. Of course, nature would provide what we need to survive.

## Stress Recovery for Your Stress Type

Considering that the research currently available shows an improvement in stress levels from all the stress recovery activities covered in this chapter, they are *all* good options for *all* the stress types! It's a matter of carefully choosing the amount and time of day to match what you need.

In the near future, I hope to see studies that show us how activities benefit different stress types specifically, and at various times of day. In the meantime, keep in mind that these stress recovery activities appear to work by helping us get out of stress mode and closer to resiliency. This means that integrating stress recovery activities into your daily schedule will help no matter what phase of the Stress Recovery Protocol you're in. They serve the purpose of bringing you back to a healthy baseline of cortisol and adrenaline.

### Stress Magnet

You should take part in stress recovery activities when your cortisol is high. If you wake up with high cortisol, that's the perfect time to meditate, journal, or spend time in nature. If your cortisol starts to rise at midday, plan a break for at least fifteen minutes to take some deep breaths, listen to music, or call a friend. Knowing your pattern can help you give your body what it needs, and when it needs it most. I know it can feel like you can't possibly fit one more activity into your day, so start with a few minutes of "you time," and remind yourself that taking breaks has been shown to improve productivity.

### Night Owl

Your cortisol increases in the evening, so you should focus on stress recovery activities at night. Make an extra effort to turn down the lights and turn on a progressive relaxation meditation. Your body needs a stronger anti-stress signal in the evening to let it know that you don't need more cortisol before bed. You may want to try journaling and/or biofeedback and measuring your heart rate variability to see the difference they make in turning off your sympathetic nervous system. Turn on calming, healing music and let your mind drift to sleep.

### Sluggish and Stressed

Having high cortisol with low adrenaline means you are a perfect candidate for stress reduction. You may find that you absolutely love meditation and yoga, because they provide a much-needed break for your body from all the cortisol. The challenge is that low adrenaline can cause you to have low stamina. If you get exhausted from your chosen activity, it just means you need to choose a shorter amount of time and perhaps something less strenuous to start with. Instead of raking all the leaves in the yard, start by picking the dead leaves off your plants and giving them water. Notice the leaves and how the plants respond to light. Be present in the moment without imposing expectations on yourself. Watch and listen to the birds outside or put on music that makes you feel good.

## Blah and Blue

Even though your cortisol is way low, don't worry: stress recovery activities won't make it go lower. In your case, they will help your adrenal glands heal and recover, plus enable them to produce more cortisol and adrenaline. It doesn't help to overdo anything, including stress reduction, when your body is already drained. So start with small increments of gentle stress reduction. Don't start with Bikram yoga or an hour of gardening. That will likely make you feel like you need to sleep for a day (or two). Pace yourself. Ten minutes may be all you can do to start. Know that your body and adrenals are healing. Yes, they can recover function. I've seen it many times before. As you start to feel better, it can be tempting to want to do more. I'm warning you because it will happen for you, too. And as you do feel better, you'll overdo it and then feel worse again. That is your body teaching you its limits. Listen to your body. It will guide you to know the types of activities and amounts that are just right, but not too much.

## Tired and Wired

Your cortisol is low in the morning and your adrenaline is high, but don't let this confuse you. These stress recovery techniques will help you, just the same. Your body will know what to do once you find the activities that feel best to you. I think you may want to start out more slowly, with five to ten minutes of the chosen activity, and if you feel your heartbeat race, then take a few nice deep breaths and stop for now. You can try again later. Choose an activity that involves silence, such as meditation, prayer, or deep breathing. Add in biofeedback if you'd like to help teach your body how to get back into parasympathetic mode more easily. As you become confident with helping your body with stressful moments, you'll be able to choose more exciting activities, such as dancing and sauna therapy.

9

# *E* for Exercise

To support adrenal stress recovery, you need to exercise at the right intensity, for the right amount of time. If you push yourself too hard and too often—or, conversely, not often enough—you risk exacerbating adrenal distress. The right formula is a matter of exercising in moderation and matching your exercise to your body and stress type. In this chapter, we will explore the influence that exercise has on all bodies and specific stress types, as well as how to create a plan that helps you to exercise while you recover from adrenal distress and to find fitness options that work for you.

## Stress and Exercise

Studies show that men and women who exercise regularly respond better under stress than those who don't exercise at all.[1] This means that if you exercise regularly, you won't feel as stressed when a stress comes along, such as a deadline at work or an issue with your parent or child. Your heart rate won't go up as much and neither will your cortisol. You'll be able to do what needs to get done, without disrupting the way you feel, or your digestion or hormones, as much. This is why exercise is considered to be one of the best activities for helping us manage stress.

7

At the same time, it's important not to overdo it! Overexercising can be a stress and can cause a sustained increase in your cortisol level. Studies show that both aerobic training and resistance (weight) training increase cortisol for up to two and a half hours after exercising, and more so after intense, prolonged exercise (more than thirty minutes). For endurance athletes, exercising at a high intensity every day, cortisol remains elevated.[2] This becomes an issue because the body doesn't have a chance to recover and repair, increasing risk of injuries and health issues, as we've discussed occurs with adrenal distress.

Overall, it is important to get the right intensity of exercise, and at the right time of day, for your body.[3] For example, aerobic exercise causes an increase in the cortisol awakening response (CAR) in adults.[4] This could be a good thing for Blah and Blue and Tired and Wired types, who tend to have a low CAR. This is not ideal for Stress Magnet and Sluggish and Stressed types, who likely have an overresponsive CAR. Exercise intensity is also a factor in that high intensity tends to increase cortisol, while low intensity decreases cortisol.[5]

What this means is that Blah and Blue, as well as Tired and Wired, should start with a small amount of exercise, such as ten to fifteen minutes. Exercising in the morning will help your cortisol and CAR improve. For Stress Magnets and Sluggish and Stressed, on the other hand, it is important to ask yourself if your exercise is too intense or for too long, and whether it could be causing your cortisol to be too high. It could benefit your health to cut back a bit.

In the case of Night Owls, if you've been exercising for long periods of time—for example, taking long runs—this could be contributing to high cortisol at night. If you haven't been exercising much, you may find that adding a small workout in the morning could help, particularly if you wake up tired. Then your body will have time to recover after your workouts, and there will be enough time for cortisol to drop before getting ready to sleep in the evening.

Trying a new routine can take some getting used to, but by listening to your body and giving it just what it needs, you'll feel better than you do now. As much as you may love the feeling of a long workout, or of not exercising at all, it's likely that an amount and intensity of exercise somewhere in the middle will help you recover from stress and feel your best.

## What Exercise Is Right for You?

When it comes to exercise, there are so many different options. It's important to do what you enjoy and look forward to doing. In this way, exercise also becomes a hobby, an activity that connects you with other people, and potentially a challenge for your mind as much as for your muscles. When asked why they don't exercise, many patients tell me it's because they don't want to go to the gym. Another common answer is that they don't have time.

Bored with your current form of exercise? Maybe it's time to switch or to try something new. Sometimes there may be activities you haven't even thought of as exercise. In my opinion, anything that raises your heart rate and causes you to use your muscles, even a little bit, is exercise. Around my house, vacuuming, cleaning, scooping litter boxes, carrying laundry, and gardening are all forms of exercise that require bending, squatting, lifting, turning, balance, and movement. Are you doing exercise that you didn't realize was exercise?

At the same time, there may be certain exercises that are better for your stress type. For example, I recommend Pilates early in the day for a Night Owl, because it takes so much focus and intensity that they feel like they've really accomplished a meaningful task and will be ready to sleep at night. Night Owls are plagued by feeling they've left things unfinished, so a solid exercise routine can help counterbalance that. For Sluggish and Stressed, a ten-minute low-impact interval training (LIIT) or high-intensity interval training (HIIT) workout in the morning may be their best option, to help reestablish their CAR, but without exhausting them too much.

## Best Exercise Options for Adrenal Support

Try taking a walk.

Although we often avoid walking in our daily lives, it is one of the simplest forms of exercise and can be a great way to start moving. Whether walking your dog, walking around the block, or walking to the store (instead of driving), the act can increase your heart rate and require you to use your muscles. Walking is considered weight-bearing exercise, which improves bone density (and prevents bone loss).[6] When I travel, I'm always amazed at how far I can walk around a city I'm exploring without even realizing the distance I've covered. Please be mindful, however, that you don't have to go long distances. In fact, it's often better to take a shorter walk and then do some stretching and core strengthening to give your muscles more attention and balance out your exercise experience.

You might prefer to take a run. Studies have shown that both men and women who run regularly have an increased life expectancy, improved mood and sleep, as well as heart and brain health. Just be careful, and be mindful that running long distances can be a stress on your body and increase risk of injuries. Stay hydrated, bring energy shots, and I encourage you to meet with a physical therapist regularly so they can give you exercises and stretches to prevent injuries. Keep in mind, too, that running long distances has been shown to increase cortisol, which can decrease other hormones and disrupt the digestion, neurotransmitters, and immune system. While recovering from adrenal distress, you may need to switch to a different form of exercise.[7]

Using the stairs is another way to get moving. We are accustomed to using an elevator every chance we get, but what if you take the stairs? In the two weeks that I lived in an apartment in St. Petersburg, Russia, I walked up and down five flights of stairs, and wouldn't you know, I was in way better shape by the time I left. Stairs raise your heart rate and cause you to use different muscles than walking or running. One study showed improved cardiovascular function from climbing three flights of stairs, three times per day, three days per week.[8] If you don't have stairs, you can use a stair-climbing machine at a gym.

No matter which exercise you choose, stretching is an important addition. While it's tempting to skip, stretching can bring a lot of relaxation, especially when you take deep breaths. In fact, when we stretch, we release endorphins, which are the feel-good hormones that are also released with many types of exercise. Stretching is important, especially if you have hypermobile joints, like I do. At the same time, you don't want to stretch too far, either. Be mindful of your body and your joints, and don't overdo it. A nice gentle stretch, while seated or standing, can be a terrific way to improve flexibility, balance, and prevent injuries.[9]

Yoga takes stretching to the next level. Yoga reduces stress, as we talked about in chapter eight, and involves intentional poses performed in a sequence while mindfully focusing on self-awareness and breath. Studies demonstrate improved strength and flexibility, cardiovascular function, mood and sleep, as well as decreased pain.[10] Many yoga classes last an hour, or more with meditation. This can be too long if you're just getting started or if you're Blah and Blue or Tired and Wired. Plan on taking breaks, which most yoga instructors will support, especially if you give them a heads-up. Or find an online yoga class that lasts ten to fifteen minutes. For me, that's the perfect amount.

Pilates is often grouped with yoga, but they are actually quite different. Pilates was developed by Joseph Pilates (along with his wife, Clara) over the course of his lifetime until he died in 1967. He was born in Germany and brought his method to the US in 1926. Joe (as he was called) was a boxer and gymnast and believed that many illnesses could be alleviated by using his method. Many world-famous people, including dancers, actors, musicians, and athletes, went to Joe's gym in New York City to keep themselves in the best shape possible.

Pilates invented special equipment that uses spring tension to develop strength, stretch, and control. He created platforms with bars and springs, one called a "Cadillac" and another called a "reformer," that allow a participant to exercise while lying down because he believed that was the best way to connect the mind to the body. I started doing Pilates seven years ago, and it has become a part of my life. It requires so much of my attention that it is like a mindfulness exercise. I pay attention to my posture while moving in small, precise movements. It's amazing how much my strength and posture have improved with Pilates. To ensure safety and effectiveness, it's important to work with a teacher who has been trained and certified. Pilates is offered in private or group classes, in person or online.[11]

Dance of all types is surely exercise, as it raises the heart rate and requires the muscles to engage. As I mentioned, I grew up performing and competing as a dancer. I find dance creative and fun. It's never the same thing twice. You can turn on the music right now and start moving, and that would be dance. Or you can sign up for ballroom dancing classes or a type of exercise based on dance, like Zumba. Dance is known to improve strength and endurance.[12] Be mindful, once again, that it's possible to overdo it here, so start with fifteen minutes or so, stay hydrated, and be sure to stretch afterwards.

Tai Chi and Qigong are ancient forms of movement in Chinese medicine. Based on an ancient martial art, Tai Chi is essentially a moving meditation involving mindfulness, rhythmic breathing, and coordination. It builds concentration, patience, and balance while also building strength. Qigong puts more emphasis on moving energy (chi) using intention, and functions as a spiritual practice as well. They are both low-impact, slow-movement exercises, so they are great places to start if you want or need to take it easy. In fact, they have been studied as a form of rehabilitation and stress management. No equipment is needed. You can start by observing a class in person or on YouTube.[13]

In weight training, the focus is on increasing muscle strength using resistance training as opposed to aerobic training. Strength is incredibly important for maintaining bone density and is also known to improve insulin function and prevent cardiovascular disease as well as cancer.[14] A person could spend hours each day preparing, lifting, and recovering. At the same time, it's possible to attain the benefits by lifting weights in short circuits, with eight to ten repetitions, and repeat that for three or four sets, depending on the weight used and the goal. I started weight training when I was in high school and loved the effect it had on my body. For me, building strength helps keep my hypermobile joints in place. At the same time, I have to be careful not to go too high with the weight, or I'll pull my joints out of place, and believe me, that's painful. I encourage you to work with a trainer who can help you know which exercises to do and what weight is best for you. Always listen to your body.

You might also prefer a strengthening workout without weights, such as abdominal or core strengthening. This is considered low-impact strength training and may involve ten to twenty minutes of ab crunches, leg lifts, squats, and lunges. These isolated movements without weights make injury less likely while also building muscle and improving balance, both of which help with stress resiliency, as well as blood sugar optimization and bone health. These low-impact exercises are perfect for anyone, but are especially helpful for Blah and Blue types whose energy is too low for high intensity and for Stress Magnets who need a workout that doesn't raise cortisol too high. Look for low-impact workouts on YouTube.

A HIIT or LIIT workout is a newer way of working out in a short period of time. I love it! High-intensity interval training (HIIT) and low-intensity interval training (LIIT) involve movements that get your heart rate up and build strength at the same time. A HIIT or LIIT workout commonly lasts for ten to fifteen minutes, which makes it easy to fit into a busy day, and also prevents you from doing too much. For every minute, you'll work hard for about thirty seconds and rest for thirty seconds. HIIT often involves full-body movements, such as burpees or swinging a kettlebell. Just be careful not to injure yourself. Always listen to your body and don't overdo it. By exercising in this way, you burn more calories, for longer, and for up to forty-eight hours after a workout. If you like the idea of efficiency and a concerted effort for a short amount of time, try a HIIT or LIIT workout, which you can find on YouTube; most trainers can also guide you through a routine.

Cycling is another type of exercise that many of my clients enjoy. After going to high school in the bicycling capital of the Northwest (Redmond, Washington), I enjoy my café bike (a road bike with flat handlebars) for casually riding around a lake and spending time in nature. For some, cycling is more of a sport and hobby, and they prep for road races or triathlons. My sister, a mother of three young girls, loves her Peloton bike, which she can ride from home. One of my patients with diabetes got her blood sugar back to normal by going to spin classes. I'm so inspired by her! There are many ways to cycle, and all are exercise. Start with a small amount of intensity and duration, increase from there, and notice how your body responds and adapts. Be careful, and wear a helmet when cycling outdoors.

There are many other forms of exercise—more than I can mention here. Swimming, hiking, and playing basketball (or any other sport) are all examples. I encourage you to choose what helps you look forward to exercising, while also allowing you to stay safe by avoiding injuries. You can also bring daily spirituality into exercise by exercising outdoors (earth), getting yourself to sweat (fire), drinking plenty of water to stay hydrated (water), and paying attention to your breathing (air).

## Getting Started with a New Routine and Monitoring Progress

I encourage you to start any new exercise routine in a thoughtful and moderate way.

An important way to monitor your exercise tolerance is by checking your heart rate. To do this, find your pulse on the thumb side of your wrist using your first two fingers (not your thumb). Count for thirty seconds and multiply by 2, or count for six seconds and multiply by 10, to get your heart rate for one minute. The target heart rate is the rate you are aiming for, to get the most benefit from exercising. For many years, exercise physiologists started by calculating maximum heart rate (by subtracting a person's age from 220), and then used a percentage to determine target heart rate depending on the intensity of the activity. More recent research, however, has shown that it is better to exercise at our maximum aerobic function (MAF), which accounts for fitness as well as nutrition and stress; this allows us to exercise at the optimal intensity for improving health while burning fat and preventing injury. To determine your MAF, subtract your age from 180. Modify this by subtracting 5 or 10 from that number if you are injured, are recovering from illness, get frequent allergy symptoms or colds, or are just starting to exercise regularly (5 if your symptoms are less severe, 10 if more severe). If you're forty years old, your MAF is 180 minus 40, or 140 beats per minute—that's what you are aiming for when you work out.

Your resting heart rate is how many times your heart beats in a minute when you are at rest and not exercising. Check this when you wake up in the morning and before you get out of bed. It's commonly between 60 and 100 beats per minute. Having a lower resting heart rate is considered more optimal. Your resting heart rate is affected by adrenaline, stress, and medications, as well as how much you exercise. Getting to know your resting heart rate will help you know your body and how it responds as you start to exercise.

Heart rate variability (HRV), which we talked about in earlier chapters, is a way of monitoring how well your heart responds to stress and recovers. As you exercise more consistently, checking your HRV can also be a good way for you to observe the benefits of exercising. You can do this with a device such as a chest band, wristband, or finger sensor.

By checking your resting heart rate and HRV, you'll be able to tell when your body is ready for more exercise. You'll also know by how you feel after a workout. If you are exhausted and feel like you need to sleep the rest of the day, you overdid it. If you are so sore that you can barely move, that was too much exercise, too. Too much movement is not the point or ultimate goal. The saying "no pain, no gain" is not true. We are rewriting the goal for exercise. The goal is to move, even a small amount, as much as feels good and isn't too much of a stress for your body. Then increase gradually, monitoring how your body responds. And if you feel worse, decrease how much and how intensely you're moving, all while allowing your body to recover and adapt.

## Exercise Routines for Your Stress Type

### Stress Magnet

Take it easy. While, yes, exercising is a good way to relieve your stress, doing too much will work against you. Aim for ten to fifteen minutes of getting your heart rate up each day. If you tend to have high cortisol in the morning, wait until midday to exercise, but don't do it too late, either. You may actually find that you'll prefer two sessions of fifteen minutes each at different times of day. Stretching or yoga could be one session, and a HIIT workout could be the other.

### Night Owl

The main thing for you is not to exercise in the evening, because it could increase your cortisol more at night, which could prevent you from falling asleep. And it would be better to exercise in the morning, to help reset your circadian rhythm and give you a boost of cortisol at the right time of day. Getting outside in the morning light will also help reset your sleep-wake cycle. Maybe go for a fifteen-minute walk or swim. If you are exhausted from not sleeping, you may need to start with five minutes of gentle movement. Don't push it. Take it one day at a time and gradually your body will shift your cortisol output so that it is stronger in the morning than in the evening.

### Sluggish and Stressed

As with the Stress Magnet, a ten- to fifteen-minute workout at midday—not when your cortisol is already high—would be perfect for you. This could be walking up a hill or stairs or using an elliptical trainer at the gym. If you want to do more, combine gentle stretching or yoga with a LIIT workout, so that you'll feel like you did more, without raising your cortisol too much. You'll know when you're ready for more when you don't feel worse the next day.

### Blah and Blue

While your energy is likely low and exercising may feel impossible, please know that you don't need to start exercise immediately. Start supporting the calming part of your nervous system in Phase 1 of the Stress Recovery Protocol and get the other aspects of C.A.R.E. going. You'll know when your body is ready to exercise. You'll start thinking about how you'd like to move, and the next thing you know, you'll choose a type of exercise that feels right. It may then be tempting to do too much, so stick to ten or fifteen minutes, and notice how you feel the next day. Start with relatively gentle exercise that adds strength and can be modified to your needs, such as Pilates or low-impact strengthening.

## Tired and Wired

Your adrenaline levels are going to give you a boost of energy and make you feel like you want to move; however, your low cortisol levels tell me you may lose steam quickly. Start with a short workout and a nice, gentle exercise in the morning, like a bike ride or walk, so you can begin to gauge your true exercise potential and not just the adrenaline pushing you through. Then, as your cortisol level improves, go for longer (but not too long!) or more intense exercise classes or strength-training workouts.

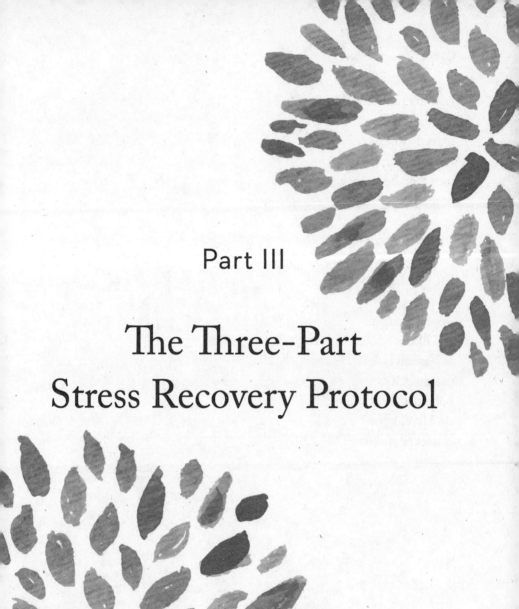

Part III

# The Three-Part
# Stress Recovery Protocol

# Phase 1 | Getting Out of Stress Mode

In part one we explored what burnout and adrenal distress are. Once there, though, how do we get out of these states? Once you know your stress type from the self-assessment in chapter four, it's a matter of using the right tools, in a strategic process, to bring your body back into balance. This includes implementing the C.A.R.E. method covered in part two, along with natural approaches to rebalance what was thrown out of balance by stress. It's a process that prioritizes your body's stress recovery above all else. If you don't approach it correctly, however, you could make it worse. One person's yoga is another person's nightmare.

As a midwife, I find that labor—the process women's bodies go through to deliver a baby—is an example for how many processes in our bodies work. First there is a preparation phase in which the body gets ready. Second is the phase when the baby is born. Third is when the placenta, which has sustained the baby through pregnancy, is delivered. It is an amazing and beautiful process that our bodies know how to do naturally. It has a beginning, middle, and end, and it leaves us ready to move forward. We don't need to teach our bodies how to deliver a baby, and we don't have to teach our bodies how to recover from stress either. We simply need to provide the right environment and support, and our bodies will heal.

In this chapter, I'll introduce you to the three phases of my Stress Recovery Protocol, individualized for each stress type. First, however, I want to guide you in establishing a stress recovery mindset, which is essential for turning burnout into stress resilience.

Success relies on identifying and changing the behaviors that contributed to your adrenal distress. I know it's tempting to want to go back to how things were before you started feeling awful. I understand that it can be scary to think that your body has limits or that you won't be able to get as much done as you used to. Please don't allow these fears to stop you from learning from your body. Stress recovery is the perfect time to learn what your body needs in order to recover and stay healthy going forward. During this process, you'll discover what was missing previously and what caused you to fall victim to stress. Gradually, as you recover, you'll have an opportunity to understand yourself and your body in a new way, and to understand the signals your body gives when it needs a break—before you end up in stress mode again.

## Claim a Stress Recovery Mindset

First, you need to get into a mindset that allows for burnout recovery. As the saying goes, you can't pour from an empty cup. To recognize how full your own cup is, I challenge you to revisit your quiz results (or do the Stress Type Quiz online) and reflect on times when you haven't been eating well or your sleep has been off. Perhaps you snapped at someone? Felt nauseated or bloated? Or had brain fog or headaches day after day?

All these seemingly isolated events tell you that stress has built up in your body and that you haven't had enough anti-stress time. This leaves you unable to be the best version of yourself. But choosing to take care of yourself can be harder than it sounds. I've personally struggled between what I learned in childhood—don't be selfish, think about others—and what I know as a doctor: putting yourself first is the key to healing and stress recovery.

If up to this point in your life, you've been an expert in serving others, making sure they have what they need, and ensuring that they are happy with what you are doing, then switching over to a "take care of me first" mindset is not as easy as it sounds. You may have experienced feelings of shame or unworthiness. Instead of thinking of what you need to do to make yourself better, you'd start thinking of all the things you need to do or what others are wanting you to do. You may have even experienced dark, convoluted thoughts that whisper, "I'm not worth it."

The reality is that you are worth it. We are not equipped to take care of others until we first acknowledge, prioritize, and have compassion for ourselves.

I have personally battled with these feelings. I pushed myself aside for over twenty years, ignoring signs of stress that manifested as severe migraines, which caused me to be in bed for days. I suffered in silence because as a naturopathic doctor I was ashamed of not being able to stop the migraines. Meanwhile, I was working to help thousands of people successfully solve their health issues, including migraines. The irony is that the migraines were my body's way of telling me I was overworked and needed to recover.

This self-sabotaging stigma is not new. The belief that we should stop focusing on ourselves and be able to keep up with life's demands without a "sick" day is terrible for our health. That's the message I grew up hearing. I recently looked at my elementary school report card and saw that I had zero missed days of school, as if that were a good thing!

Finally, I stopped running long enough to figure out that if I planned stress recovery time, my body wouldn't have to force time off by having a migraine—and that's when everything changed. It became my priority to set up the perfect work schedule, with breaks and time to exercise and de-stress. I looked for every opportunity to support my body through each workday and blocked out time to not work (imagine that!). It was the first time in over twenty years that I made Saturday a weekend day, not a workday. I got a standing desk so I could maintain good posture while at my computer. And I set my schedule so that I could meditate, exercise, and have a nutritious meal before starting appointments and meetings for the day.

You can do all of this, too. To be successful, though, you need to first understand the three critical aspects of a stress recovery mindset: awareness, accountability, and willingness to create change.

## Become Aware of What Needs to Change

The reticular activating system (RAS) is a part of our brain that sorts through (subconscious) information and determines which thoughts or emotions to bring to our conscious awareness. The default for how the RAS determines which information to prioritize is to "look for" what it recognizes from our past. This is why we tend to find ourselves repeating patterns and re-creating scenarios (even unpleasant experiences) in our lives, without our realizing it.

As that happens, cortisol and adrenaline respond in the same way, based on our genetics and epigenetics. When we allow our past to be the default for the RAS, it's no wonder we find ourselves in the same (or similar) frustrating, stressful situations. But there is another option!

If, on the other hand, we use our conscious mind to intentionally put the focus on something different, we can direct our RAS to look for something that will lead us toward a desired outcome. We automatically start doing things differently, shifting our schedule, buying different foods, and choosing different activities. Have you ever noticed a certain type of car, and then suddenly it seems like you see that same car everywhere you look? That's because your brain is finding what you signaled it to look for. With practice and consistency, our brain will guide us toward what we want with ease.

Instead of re-creating stress, which ultimately leads to burnout, you can tell your brain to create balance. And as you do, little by little, day by day, it becomes more likely that your brain will automatically guide you to a new normal. It will become easier to choose relaxation. It will become second nature to buy arugula and flaxseed oil at the store, instead of packaged foods and canola oil. Once you have trained your RAS what you'd like to create in your future, instead of simply re-creating the past, it won't feel so difficult to make changes.

It can also help to remember that you are living in a human body with a built-in stress response system. That system can kick into survival mode and create a perpetual state of fear that traps you and even makes you afraid to be out of survival mode. Notice that you are not the fear. You are the person living in this human body, and you can choose what you want to focus on in any moment. Will you allow fear to run your life? Or will you find a way to choose stress recovery?

This is important to understand and implement when it comes to stress and adrenal distress recovery. Otherwise, you might make short-term changes that last for only a short period of time, until your subconscious mind takes over again. The next thing you know, you're back where you started. That's what the term *falling off the wagon* refers to: the tendency to revert back to a prior pattern. Change requires that you become completely clear about what you'd like to experience going forward and disciplined about creating it. Giving yourself personalized support based on your stress type will allow you to live your best life.

## Get to Know the Phases of the Stress Recovery Protocol

I developed my stress recovery approach over years of helping patients and myself recover from burnout. I've seen what doesn't work, and I've identified the pitfalls that can send you straight back to burnout. Now that I've figured out the essential steps, and the order to implement them, I want to share that information, so you know how to get out of stress mode, optimize your cortisol and adrenaline levels, and cure your stress once and for all.

Before describing how each stress type can implement the Stress Recovery Protocol, I want to first describe the overall phases, so that you have the big-picture concept in mind. Then we'll talk it through from the perspective of how each stress type can achieve recovery. There are three phases of the Stress Recovery Protocol:

- Phase 1. Calm: Get out of stress mode with calming support and by reducing stress exposure. Emphasis on connection with yourself.
- Phase 2. Balance: Optimize cortisol, adrenaline levels, and more. Continue to connect with yourself as you become more confident connecting with others.
- Phase 3. Resilience: Maintain resilience to stress. Keeping balance within yourself while exploring more of the world around you.

The first two phases restore healthy levels of cortisol, adrenaline, and neurotransmitters. At the same time, it's important to optimize the digestion (heal leaky gut and rebalance gut bacteria), decrease inflammation, and support healthy hormone levels. In this way, you are correcting the imbalances stress caused. As you rebalance your levels, you'll become more resilient to any stresses that come along. Optimal levels will also make it easier to process the emotions associated with past stresses and to make deeper connections with people in your life.

Once everything is balanced, you'll also know what your body needs to maintain those levels over time, which brings us to phase three. Maintaining optimal levels doesn't usually require the same amount of effort and supplements as is needed when you are depleted. It does require that you use your newfound connection with yourself and awareness for how stress affects you to feel confident interacting in the world without fear of returning to stress mode. Even so, once you've completed the protocol, you'll know which nutrients, herbs, and activities to turn to when you are under more stress.

## Stress Recovery Protocol

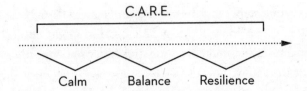

## Using Nutrients and Herbs to Restore Health

I first took biochemistry when I was a college student, specifically studying its role in nutrition and science. I was amazed. To realize that we can break down every process in our bodies into sequential steps and that our bodies inherently know how to run these steps every day is mind-blowing. Then in naturopathic medical school I studied biochemistry (again), as well as clinical nutrition (use of nutrients for health concerns) and herbal medicine (how herbs work and when to use each of them).

You don't need to take a biochemistry class or an herbalism course to benefit from them. I'm going to guide you on how to give your body the nutrients and herbs it needs to reestablish healthy levels of neurotransmitters, hormones, and more. Using nutrients—such as vitamins, minerals, and amino acids—we are essentially giving your body what it needs to run the processes it already knows how to do. But we need the right nutrients, in optimal amounts, for it to work. Same with plant medicine—we want to use the plant shown to cause the effect your body needs.

When it comes to balancing neurotransmitters, we are going to use amino acids because they are the precursor nutrient (the body turns amino acids into neurotransmitters). Amino acids come from protein in our diet. If you were to break protein down to its tiniest parts, you'd be looking at amino acids. There are twenty amino acids used in the human body for various purposes, including building muscles, detoxification processes, and making adrenaline and neurotransmitters.

We can make eleven of the twenty amino acids within our bodies. The other nine we must get from food. In our diet, it is best to consume a combination of amino acids so we have enough of each (which is why it is important to choose complete protein sources). However, in clinical nutrition, we can provide a specific amino acid in order to increase the production of the substance made from that amino acid. Targeted amino acid therapy (TAAT) is the term used to describe the use of amino acids to balance neurotransmitters.[1] I have been using TAAT for over twenty years with great success.

What I want you to know is that it is possible to address neurotransmitter (brain chemical) imbalances using nutrients. And it is possible to give your adrenal glands the nutrients and herbs they need to restore healthy production of cortisol and adrenaline, just as it is possible to give your intestinal cells the nutrients and herbs they need to recover from leaky gut.

## Phase 1: Use Calming Support to Get Out of Stress Mode

We have to start with calming support. When you feel tired and burned-out, it's so tempting to give yourself a boost of energy. But if you stimulate yourself more, without having enough calm to counterbalance, that will only work against you. It's like pressing the gas pedal when you don't have brakes. You're likely to aggravate your anxiety, sleep issues, and worries. Why do that to yourself when there's another way that doesn't have to involve feeling worse?

Instead, we start with calming, as it's only once you are out of stress mode that your body can truly heal. That means increasing calming neurotransmitters, decreasing cortisol and adrenaline if they are high, and generally giving your body the signal that it doesn't need to be reacting to stress. We want to overemphasize safety, predictability, and consistency each and every day (and night), giving your body the fewest possible reasons to jump back into stress mode. Again, that's why establishing a connection with yourself and a self-care routine is so important.

Phase 1 is the perfect time to decrease your stress exposure, especially in terms of avoiding toxins, inflammatory foods and food sensitivities (discussed in chapter six), lack of sleep, and overexercising. That's where C.A.R.E. comes in: it's how you ensure you're not sending yourself right back into stress mode.

It is also the time to make space in your daily schedule for you. I call it a "daily check-in" where each day you assess your energy, mood, focus, sleep, and how you feel in your body. Notice how many hours of sleep, stress recovery, and exercise you got. And how do you feel? Are there any anxieties or insecurities coming up? If so, be present with yourself in a loving way and give yourself compassionate support to know everything will be okay.

Phase 1 can take anywhere from days to weeks to months. It depends on your body and your ability to implement these changes in your life. Stress mode causes some people to react to every single thing, even things that are good for them. It can seem like every change, even good changes, makes things worse. If this is the case for you, you'll need to approach stress mode with the greatest amount of stealth and suavity. You'll need to start with the tiniest changes and give yourself a lot of positive feedback and mantras to keep moving forward on this path.

It can help to remember that healing is not a straightforward or overnight process, but more of a two-steps-forward and one-step-back process. So be patient with yourself. As one patient explained, "When you've been going 140 miles an hour every day, the gas pedal is always accelerating, so you no longer know what slowing down feels like, and it can feel scary or strange." You won't know if today is going to be full of taking steps forward or backward. You'll need to be able to maintain curiosity about what's happening in your body while also keeping steady with your intention and mindset. Remind yourself that every step along the way is a learning opportunity.

Try noticing your thoughts, feelings, symptoms, and experiences, but not being attached or reactive to them (as with meditation). Allow your experience to simply be what it is. And at the same time, be totally committed to the process of feeling better, getting out of stress mode, and recovering from stress so that you can feel your best and live your passion and purpose.

Phase 1 looks different for each person, though it always involves getting out of stress mode. For dogs, it might look like a shake. They shake, and the stress is gone. For us, as humans, it's not as easy. Like a spring that's sprung, your body needs to get back to a ready position.

For Stress Magnets and Night Owls, this phase is focused on decreasing cortisol and adrenaline during their elevated times of day. Tired and Wireds need their adrenaline to drop down to optimal. All of the stress types, including Blah and Blue, need to support their calming neurotransmitters, which have likely been depleted by stress. Having enough calming support is essential before moving on to Phase 2.

Various herbs and nutrients can help you achieve equilibrium and get you out of stress mode. In Phase 1, focus particularly on nutrients, amino acid supplements, and herbal medicine to normalize your stress hormone levels and decrease inflammation by starting to heal leaky gut.

## Support Calming Neurotransmitters

GABA and Serotonin are the two main calming neurotransmitters. We can support them using amino acid precursors and GABA itself in supplement form.

### Theanine

Theanine, an amino acid found in tea leaves, is the perfect example of what we all need in Phase 1 of stress recovery. Theanine has been found to support GABA and serotonin, two of the main calming neurotransmitters.[2] Increasing these neurotransmitters promotes relaxation, sleep, and stress recovery. Plus, these neurotransmitters are often depleted by stress, so you likely need more. Theanine is known to be generally safe and gentle. Common dosing is 100 to 200 mg (and up to 400 mg) every four to six hours throughout the day, and at bedtime. Notice how you feel when you take it and adjust the dose to match what you need.

### GABA

GABA itself is available in supplement form, over the counter. While there is some controversy over how it gets into the nervous system through the blood-brain barrier, study after study and clinical cases demonstrate its effectiveness, so we know that it is working somehow. Some studies have shown that it communicates with the nervous system via bacteria in the gut. And others have indicated it may be leaking across a stressed and leaky blood-brain barrier. Either way, supporting GABA levels with actual GABA is effective for most people and does not result in any sort of dependency or withdrawal, which is known to occur with pharmaceutical medications that work by stimulating GABA receptors, such as benzodiazepines.[3] GABA may be combined with theanine, and the dose is between 200 and 500 mg, once or twice per day, and/ or before bed (if needing support with sleep).

## 5-HTP

Supporting serotonin is another way to buoy the calming part of the nervous system and help shift your body out of stress mode. Tryptophan is the precursor amino acid to serotonin. While you could use tryptophan, two reasons make it a less-than-optimal choice. First, tryptophan can go down a different pathway, to make a substance called kynurenic acid, which is a neurotoxin. And when our bodies are stressed, they are more likely to send tryptophan down this undesired pathway. Second, tryptophan has to be converted to 5-hydroxotryptophan (5-HTP) first, and then to serotonin, so it's a two-step process. However, 5-HTP itself can be used, cutting this down to a one-step process and avoiding the risk of increasing anything other than serotonin.[4] The latter is the approach that I prefer.

When supporting serotonin using 5-HTP, it is important to begin with a low dose, say 50 to 100 mg. That is because our bodies and nervous systems are used to the amount of serotonin they currently have. If we increase our serotonin too quickly, our nervous systems will notice it and may cause us to feel stimulated instead of relaxed. I refer to this as a "serotonin celebration," because the nervous system is so excited to see more serotonin show up. And the paradox is that the lower our serotonin level is to start with, the more likely we are to experience a serotonin celebration when we introduce 5-HTP.

For this reason, I encourage you to start with a low dose of this supplement, taken during the day and with food, to get a sense of how your body responds to 5-HTP. After about a week of taking it, you'll likely find that your nervous system is used it. You'll be able to increase the dose if desired, and move the dose to bedtime, because it can help you to feel more relaxed and to sleep more deeply. The doses I commonly find to be effective are between 100 and 200 mg per day. Some people prefer to take this supplement in the morning. You really have to see how you feel and find the best timing and dose for you.

Although 5-HTP is generally safe, if you are taking a medication that affects the serotonin receptors, such as an SSRI or SNRI, it is extremely important to work with a practitioner who is trained in the use of amino acids. This is because when you are taking a medication that blocks the breakdown of serotonin and you take 5-HTP to increase serotonin production, you could end up with too much serotonin—a condition known as serotonin syndrome.

## Decrease Cortisol When Elevated

The other major players with stress mode are cortisol and adrenaline. We need to make sure they are not elevated, at any point during the day, in order to get you out of stress mode.

### Phosphatidylserine

Phosphatidylserine (PS) is an amino acid (serine) combined with a phospholipid produced within our bodies that has been shown to decrease production of cortisol.[5] It does this by resetting the cortisol receptors in the hypothalamus, which can get stuck in the "on mode" when we are exposed to chronic stress.

PS actually exists throughout the human brain and is involved in memory and cognition. Although we can make it, we get most of it from our food, such as from soy products and egg yolks. It's safe to take as a supplement and is considered a nootropic, a substance that improves cognitive function.

Between 500 and 1,500 mg once or twice per day will decrease cortisol when it's too high. While sometimes it can be dosed morning and night, I prefer to dose it near the time of day when cortisol is too high, so that it can be used to reset cortisol exactly when needed. I encourage patients to start with a low dose, get to know how their body responds, and then increase the dose if needed, until they find that their cortisol levels start shifting in the right direction. They'll know because they'll feel less stressed and be more likely to fall asleep at a desired bedtime and stay asleep all night.

### Herbs to Decrease Cortisol

Numerous herbs have been shown to help decrease cortisol that is too high. Many times, I see these herbs used in general stress formulas, even without knowing that your cortisol is too high. This is because herbs tend to be adaptogenic, which means they help bring the body back to a balance point, whether cortisol levels are too far gone in one direction or the other. I prefer to use herbs in doses that have a more definite effect, so that is the information I'm providing here.

Ashwagandha (*Withania somnifera*) is perhaps the most well-known herb to address cortisol levels. While studies have shown it helps optimize cortisol in general, the most definitive studies indicate that it is best at lowering cortisol that is too high.[6] We don't yet know the exact mechanism of action, but I believe it works by causing the hypothalamic receptors to be more responsive to cortisol, thus inhibiting the production of cortisol when there is plenty of it in the bloodstream. Common dosing is 250 to 500 mg once or twice per day. While many patients report to me that they have experienced great benefit from the use of ashwagandha, I find it to be mildly effective. It is known to be a nightshade, which means that those who feel worse when consuming nightshades may not do well with ashwagandha. Otherwise, it has very few side effects and these are rare.

More clinically effective than ashwagandha are banaba leaf (*Lagerstroemia specioa*) and magnolia root (*Magnolia officinalis*). They have both been shown to decrease cortisol levels when they are elevated and, specifically, to reduce the conversion of cortisone to active cortisol.[7] Magnolia root is often combined with *Phellodendron amurense*, also known to reduce stress.

Banaba leaf or Magnolia root, or both, can be taken in a supplement form, and they can be used along with phosphatidylserine. I suggest, again, that you start at a low dose and take them at the time of day when you need to decrease your cortisol level. Increase the dose until you have the desired effect, and maintain that dose until you notice that your body has shifted out of stress mode. Then you can decrease the dose and maintain the benefit. Eventually, you can stop taking these herbs, so long as your body stays out of stress mode without them. Or you can take them as needed during a stressful period.

While rhodiola (*Rhodiola rosea*) is also used to help reset cortisol production, it's important to pay attention to the dose as rhodiola causes different responses in the body based on the dose. A very high dose of rhodiola, 576 mg containing 16 mg of rhodioloside, will decrease cortisol production, whereas a low dose will increase cortisol production (we'll discuss that in chapter 11).[8] There are not many rhodiola products available with a high enough dose to decrease cortisol, so I seldom use it for this purpose. Nonetheless, I want you to be aware of these facts because you may find rhodiola in products that are intended to decrease cortisol, but in actuality, the dose is not high enough to accomplish that. Instead, rhodiola is best used in products to increase cortisol.

## Decrease Adrenaline When Elevated

Adrenaline, as we discussed in chapter one, is a term I use for both norepinephrine and epinephrine. They are metabolized through the COMT enzyme, which is influenced by the *COMT* genes. Toxins, inflammation, and stress in general also affect the functioning of COMT, which means that when you are more stressed, you are more likely to have a higher level of adrenaline. You may also have high dopamine levels. This effect is natural and makes sense when we think about how our bodies are built to help us respond to stress and survive. Adrenaline helps us respond when we're under stress. But if your COMT is stuck in stress mode, causing your adrenaline (and possibly dopamine) to trend high more of the time, you are likely to experience anxiety and a racing heart, even when you are not stressed. In that case, you can use the nutrients vitamin C and magnesium to encourage COMT to metabolize adrenaline faster.[9]

### Magnesium

Magnesium comes in many forms: citrate, oxide, glycinate, malate, and threonate, for example. It's all about what the magnesium is attached to, and the substance it is attached to determines where it has the most effect. Citrate and oxide, for example, are most effective at encouraging regular bowel movements. Glycinate and malate signal muscles to relax. Threonate, on the other hand, signals calming in the nervous system, and it does this by supporting the function of COMT. Common doses of magnesium are between 100 and 400 mg once or twice per day. If you experience loose stools, then decrease the dose. Otherwise, magnesium is known as generally safe and can be used and dosed in a way that provides the most benefit.

### B Vitamins

B vitamins, such as vitamin B6, folate (B9), and B12, are also essential for the metabolism of dopamine and adrenaline (norepinephrine and epinephrine).

This leads us into addressing methylation, which is a complex process in itself. Methylation is the way our bodies use B vitamins to make a substance called SAM (S-adenosylmethionine), which is used for making and breaking down neurotransmitters (among many other roles in the body).

I'm mentioning B vitamins here because they are important for the metabolism of adrenaline;[10] however, I don't usually recommend adding or increasing them at the beginning of Phase 1. For some people, when they are under stress, methylation stops working well. If they increase the amount of B vitamins coming through methylation, it can make them feel worse by aggravating their anxiety and cause headaches.

I suggest you wait until you have implemented more self-care, decreased inflammation in your body, and improved the state of your gut bacteria, all of which help methylation work better. Then, and only if your labs indicate that you need them, you can consider adding B6, folate (5-MTHF), and B12 (methylcobalamin), and/or SAMe (which is SAM in a supplement form), to help manage adrenaline. I suggest finding a practitioner who understands how to optimize B vitamin doses for your body. I work very closely with patients with methylation issues and MTHFR gene variations and have created an online program available at DoctorDoni.com to help.

## Heal Leaky Gut

We spoke, in chapter six, about how having delayed food sensitivities (IgA and IgG antibody reactions) are a sign that the cells lining your intestines are not as healthy as they could be. When we are stressed, burned-out, and exposed to pesticides and medications, our bodies are not able to keep up with making enough intestinal cells to replace the damaged cells. At the same time, our food is not being digested as well, and so undigested food particles are able to leak through the intestinal walls where our immune system is on guard for foreign invaders. An immune mediated inflammatory response ensues, sending a signal of stress to your brain. If we don't put a stop to this constant source of stress from within our bodies, we won't be able to shut off stress mode. This is why it is so important to start addressing leaky gut during Phase 1 of stress recovery.

Healing leaky gut takes time. But I know it is possible to heal the gut lining because I was able to heal it myself back when I had every food sensitivity under the sun and extreme adrenal distress. Since then I've helped thousands of patients heal mild to severe leaky gut, which has given me the opportunity to see every scenario in which it presents and to try many treatment strategies. I always come from the mindset of wanting to use dietary changes, nutrients, and herbs to support the body to heal itself in the most efficient and effective way. That's how I identified my leaky gut healing protocol:

1.   Avoid the most reactive foods for you, plus gluten
2.   Support digestion of your food and regular bowel movements
3.   Provide nutrients and herbs to promote healing of intestinal cells
4.   Address imbalanced gut bacteria and optimize microbiome

I'll guide you through each step below. And if you need more help, please turn to my online programs where I guide participants to heal leaky gut in the most strategic way.

## Avoid the most reactive foods for you

Whether you do a food sensitivity test or food elimination diet to determine which foods to avoid, I want to make sure you know that the goal is not to avoid every food or too many foods. We need you to still be getting enough macronutrients and calories to maintain your weight. At the same time, to be most effective, it is important to avoid the foods that are triggering an inflammatory response because they are perpetuating leaky gut. In most cases, that means avoiding gluten, because gluten is inherently inflammatory.

## Support digestion of your food and regular bowel movements

When food is better digested, it doesn't trigger an inflammatory response or overfeed bacteria. When the intestines are able to move contents through at an optimal rate, that helps us to absorb nutrients and eliminate toxins. Stress recovery activities we discussed in chapter eight, especially those that support vagal tone, will help your body to get better at digesting food and having a daily bowel movement that is formed and complete.

Eating foods that are bitter, such as arugula, also signals to your body to turn on digestive function. I find that the patients who heal fastest also take a supplement containing pancreatic enzymes. Whether animal derived or plant derived, these enzymes (namely protease, amylase, and lipase) normally produced by the pancreas and intestinal cells are able to digest our macronutrients—protein, carbs, and fat.[11] When you take enzymes as a supplement, it does not suppress your body's ability to make them. As you recover from adrenal distress, your natural enzyme production will improve, and then you won't need to swallow enzyme support.

Drinking enough water (preferably filtered), and not too much, throughout the day, and getting electrolytes is also important for healthy digestive function. I suggest drinking 2 to 4 ounces of water (depending on your body size, activity level, and caffeine intake) every 2 to 4 hours when awake. For electrolytes, try adding a pinch of sea salt to your water (or 1 teaspoon of sea salt in a gallon of water). Sea salt contains a balance of all the minerals versus table salt, which is mainly sodium, which is why sea salt is not associated with an increase in blood pressure. If you have high blood pressure, be sure to check with your doctor and monitor your blood pressure closely.

For those of you who struggle with constipation, in addition to supporting your vagus nerve and drinking adequate amounts of water, magnesium citrate or oxide can be helpful solutions. Magnesium is essential for the muscles in the bowels to function, so it causes a bowel movement without creating a dependency, which is the case for laxative products. You can use magnesium on a daily basis if needed to maintain consistent bowel movements.

### Provide nutrients and herbs to promote healing of intestinal cells

Our bodies normally make new intestinal cells every day, so by the time we stop bombarding our intestines with inflammatory foods, and start digesting our food better, already we give our intestinal cells a better chance of catching up. While there are many nutrients and herbs that can help, I find it works best to concentrate on those that have the greatest potential for benefit and the least likelihood of overwhelming an already sensitive system. The paradox "more is not better" is true for healing leaky gut. As much as we want to heal it, if we do too much, it will backfire.

Studies show that we can help out this process with the amino acid glutamine. Glutamine is known to enhance the growth of new intestinal cells, while decreasing oxidative stress and inflammation. That is exactly what is needed! Plus glutamine improves the function of the proteins holding the intestinal cells together, called "tight junctions." These cell-to-cell connections prevent food from leaking between the cells.[12] And you don't even need a high dose of glutamine to accomplish this task. I suggest between 500 mg and 3,000 mg per day in a powder or capsule form. Collagen powder and bone broth are both sources of glutamine, which can also be helpful for healing leaky gut.

In terms of herbs, the two I turn to first for healing intestinal cells are licorice root (*Glycyrrhiza glabra*), specifically in the form deglycyrrhizinated licorice (DGL, which means they have removed the part of the root that can affect blood pressure levels), and aloe vera. Both of these herbs are known to decrease inflammation and promote healing.[13] The dosages used are 250 to 500 mg per day of DGL and 100 mg per day of aloe. I want to emphasize that it is better to begin with a lower dose and increase gradually as you assess how your body responds. As leaky gut heals, then you may be able to add additional herbs and nutrients, such as slippery elm, quercetin, and N-acetyl glucosamine, to speed up the process.

### Address imbalanced gut bacteria and optimize microbiome

This step requires that you are ready for Phase 2 of stress recovery, so I'm going to cover this in detail in chapter 11.

## Monitoring Progress and When More Help Is Needed

Optimally, you should have your cortisol, adrenaline, neurotransmitters, and food sensitivities tested prior to beginning the Stress Recovery Protocol (see chapter four). Then repeat the testing six to twelve months later to assess the effectiveness of your doses. Once you reach an optimal level, then you'll want to determine the dose that will maintain that level over time, which is influenced by your stress exposure, dietary intake of protein, and genetics. This is what I guide participants in my group programs to do so that they become masters of their own health.

If you are under a great deal of stress, you may need a prescription medication to help get you out of stress mode. Again, it's important to know your body and what it needs. Then, as you begin to feel better, a practitioner with training in using amino acids and balancing neurotransmitters can help you reoptimize your calming neurotransmitters using nutrients, and even help you understand your genetics related to processing amino acids and neurotransmitters so that, going forward, you know which nutrients, and at what dose, to take to maintain a balance under stress. This is what I do when I work with patients one-on-one.

I want to note that if you have elevated phenylalanine (PEA) and/or glutamate, you should plan to spend much more time in Phase 1, and I encourage you to reach out to a practitioner who specializes in amino acid therapy, as well as genetic variations and toxicity, because it's quite likely that you are going to need more assistance to help your body get out of stress mode. By the time that PEA and/or glutamate increase, you've been exposed to a high level of stress and trauma, and very likely nutrient deficiencies, chronic infections, and/or toxins, for a long period of time. Your body has compensated by increasing PEA and glutamate as protection mechanisms, but those protection mechanisms are working against you. It's going to require a concerted effort and detailed intervention beyond the contents of this book to help your body shift out of stress mode. What I describe here will help, and self-care is essential, but please know that your body needs more attention and that trained practitioners exist who can guide you.

## Phases of Recovery for Your Stress Type

### Stress Magnet

An example protocol is to begin Phase 1 by taking magnesium threonate to decrease adrenaline levels, and you may need to take it twice or even three times per day. Vitamin C can also help decrease adrenaline levels at 500 mg twice per day. Add in phosphatidylserine along with ashwagandha, banaba leaf, or magnolia root at the time of day when your cortisol is too high, or a few hours prior to that increase. For example, if your cortisol is higher than optimal when you wake in the morning, then you'll plan to take phosphatidylserine and banaba leaf (or another herb to decrease cortisol) upon awakening. However, you'll get the best results if you also take them before you go to bed at night, to prevent cortisol from rising too high and/or too early in the morning. If, instead, your cortisol begins to rise higher in the afternoon, right when it should be decreasing, then you'd take these supplements a few hours prior to the increase, and you might repeat the dose a few hours later.

## Night Owl

In your case, cortisol is high at night, so in Phase 1 you'll want to supplement with ashwagandha (or another herb) and phosphatidylserine in the evening and may repeat the dose at bedtime, which has been shown to help decrease cortisol production by resetting the stress signal from the brain. Start with low doses and gradually increase until you find the doses that are most effective for you. You'll know it's working when you feel more relaxed in the evening and find it easier to go to sleep and stay asleep. You will also want to take magnesium (threonate or glycinate) in the evening to prevent adrenaline from waking you.

## Sluggish and Stressed

Your cortisol is high at certain times of day, but your adrenaline is low. In Phase 1, you need to get your cortisol levels into an optimal range. Follow the same instructions as for Stress Magnet and Night Owl in terms of taking phosphatidylserine and herbs that lower cortisol, at the time of day that your levels are too high. If this is all day long, repeat your doses every three to six hours.

## Blah and Blue

Your cortisol and adrenaline levels are on the low side, but Phase 1 is not the time to address them. You'll need to first address your calming neurotransmitters (serotonin and GABA) and work on healing leaky gut. Once you have established a buffer to stress, you'll be ready to move on to Phase 2 and that is when you can support cortisol and adrenaline production.

## Tired and Wired

Those with this stress type have a bit of a tricky situation. But it's not impossible to get back on track. Just know that you'll need to pay close attention to how your body responds and adjust accordingly. First things first: decrease that adrenaline level. Your high adrenaline is your body's attempt to help you with stress, but it ends up stressing you out more. It can feel like a tight circle of anxiety and overwhelm, with underlying fatigue that leaves you unmotivated to deal with it. You've got this! Start by taking magnesium threonate to help your body process adrenaline. Vitamin C is another good nutrient for you because it improves adrenaline metabolism and adrenal recovery at the same time.

It's possible that you may have an underlying toxicity, such as mold exposure, metals (for example, from amalgam fillings in your teeth), or perhaps overgrowing gut bacteria. All these things decrease your ability to metabolize adrenaline. If you do identify toxicity, it is important to address it with the help of a practitioner who understands how not to trigger more stress in the process.

## Keep Track of How You Feel

One important point to consider while working on Phase 1 is that you're likely to still experience fatigue and possibly low motivation. Believe me, almost everyone wishes they could resolve the fatigue sooner than possible. It's tempting to want to take something to increase your energy level. But remember, if you support your energy too soon, you are liable to push yourself right back into stress mode. For now, just know that the fatigue is part of the healing process and you'll be able to address it very soon.

As you take these supplements and implement daily self-care, keep note of how you feel. When you have the dosing right, you'll start to notice that your system calms down. The racing thoughts and hypervigilance stop. The static goes away (patients often describe a feeling of static, as if the radio station is not tuned). The startle response you might be feeling disappears and you begin to feel more like "yourself"—the self you knew before you were so stressed. That's when you know you are ready for Phase 2.

# Phase 2 | Balance

## Optimize Cortisol, Adrenaline, and More

You're feeling more like yourself. You've supported your calming neurotransmitters. And you're ready to move on to the next step, which
is to support cortisol and/or adrenaline at the times of day when they
become too low and to help your adrenal glands recover from all that stress.
It's also the time to rebalance any other areas that are out of balance—whether
these are nutrients, hormones, or your digestion.

Think of it this way: In Phase 1, you developed balance at the core, calmness within, and a connection with yourself that will help you stay centered,
even when confronted with daily stresses. Now, in Phase 2, it's time to expand
that state of balance to other areas of your body and your life, to create a foundation to keep you steady under greater amounts of stress. Then, in Phase 3,
we'll build a safety net or shield of resilience around you, so you have a strat-
egy to bounce back from whatever comes your way.

I want to emphasize that the intention here is to give your body, and your
adrenal glands, what they need to heal and recover from stress, so they can
support you going forward.

If you are a Stress Magnet or Night Owl, you might not need to support cortisol and adrenaline levels. They may have corrected themselves already in Phase 1. It's also possible, and I see this often with patients, that you now have either low cortisol or low adrenaline or both (which is especially easy to know if you retest your levels) even if you didn't before Phase 1. That's because stress mode often covers up an essential deficiency. It's as though your stress type has shifted, but I don't see it that way. Stress Magnets and Night Owls, in particular, have an initial response that raises cortisol and adrenaline. As the body heals, those levels shift lower. In some cases, the shift is due to chronic inflammation that causes cortisol to transition into cortisone. As the inflammation decreases, with C.A.R.E. and Phase 1, it becomes clear that the adrenals have become depleted. At the same time, they're ready to be healed.

Another possibility is that you have a mixed stress type where perhaps you had (before Phase 1) elevated cortisol and/or adrenaline at one time of day and now you are left with low cortisol and/or adrenaline at a different time of day. For example, you might be a combination of Night Owl and Tired and Wired. In this mix, Phase 2 will focus on raising cortisol when it's low in the morning, while preventing it from going high again at night.

Once you complete Phase 2 of Stress Recovery, you'll be fully balanced and ready for homeostasis to maintain it.

## Essential Tips to Rebalance and Recover

Many nutrients and herbs have been shown to help the adrenal glands make more cortisol and adrenaline. If you think about it, adrenal function is what keeps us going. It is essential to life and survival. The foods we eat, the sleep we get, the nutrients and plants we consume, and even the bacterial balance in our intestines influence the ability of our adrenal glands to keep up with our stress exposure. I'm going to highlight some of the main nutrients and herbs I like to use, and why. Keep in mind that, as with most things, it's important to choose what works best for your body. For one person, that might be individual nutrients, and for another person, that might be herbs in combination. And for still others, it might be a combination of both nutrients and herbs, or something completely different, such as homeopathy, peptide therapy, and/or glandular hormonal support.

I encourage you to always be curious and observe how your body responds. If you don't notice a response at all, that's also important. It means you need to try a different herb or different dose or combination. If you feel overstimulated, it's important to decrease the doses or stop altogether and go back to Phase 1. There's no reason to make yourself feel worse or more stressed. At the same time, many people stop right there. They think, "This isn't working for me—I can't take adrenal support." To me, that isn't the correct observation. If you feel worse, your body is telling you that the particular product or dose or time of day isn't right. Perhaps you need more calming support before starting Phase 2. Perhaps you're allergic to one of the ingredients. Or perhaps your body is even responding to the nutrients and herbs as a stress. You need to go back and figure out which stresses still exist and resolve them before coming back to try Phase 2 again.

This was the case for me. I tried adrenal support way back when I was a medical student. Of course, I was under extreme stress. I was taking more than twenty credits per semester and staying up all night, several nights per week, while also on call delivering babies as a midwifery student. But when I took adrenal support—I believe it was an herbal tincture at the time—I felt worse. I got heart palpitations and felt more stressed. At the time I didn't know about Phase 1 (I hadn't discovered it yet!), so I gave up, thinking I couldn't take adrenal support. It wasn't until years later, after my daughter was born and I was running a nonprofit alongside my patient practice, that I tested my serotonin and GABA levels and found that they were severely depleted. Once I addressed them, I was finally able to take adrenal support and have it work for me.

By the way, if you have heart palpitations (like me), then consider taking coenzyme Q10 (CoQ10)—more on that later in this chapter.

If your cortisol and/or adrenaline are very low, I encourage you to see an endocrinologist to determine whether you actually have Addison's disease or another condition that causes such low levels. In that case, you may actually need to replace cortisol levels with an external source. This may be in the form of hydrocortisone, which is available by prescription and requires that you work with a practitioner. Even then, whenever possible, I would rather you support the healing of your adrenal glands, so they can produce the cortisol and adrenaline, than rely on an outside source (unless absolutely necessary). It is important to monitor your cortisol levels and to get more help from a practitioner if you are not seeing results or have trouble finding the best dosing. I very often find patients benefit more when they meet with me often through this part of the process.

## Support Cortisol Production

In order to understand which nutrients and herbs to take, we need to think about how the adrenal glands make cortisol in the first place. Cortisol is produced in the mitochondria of the cells in the adrenal glands. It follows, then, that to increase cortisol production, we need to support the mitochondria. Again, these are the tiny engines (often referred to as powerhouses) that turn nutrients into energy in cells throughout our bodies. With cortisol, they are involved in the steps of turning cholesterol into cortisol.

There are many ways to support mitochondria, and in fact, some of the best ways to support them are included in C.A.R.E., so you are already helping your mitochondria. Everything from eating a healthy diet, to fasting overnight, to strengthening muscles, to getting good sleep helps your mitochondria and, in turn, adrenal function.

Nutrients that support the mitochondria include CoQ10, N-acetylcysteine (NAC), the B vitamins, alpha lipoic acid (ALA), omega-3 fats, magnesium, L-carnitine, and PQQ (Pyrroloquinoline quinone). These nutrients are all involved in the processes inside the mitochondria, helping to transport nutrients in and out of mitochondria and, as antioxidants, protecting the mitochondria from stress, particularly oxidative stress.[1]

In addition to supporting mitochondria, you can support the adrenal glands themselves to produce more cortisol with:

- Vitamin C: 500 to 1,000 mg once or twice per day
- Vitamin B5 (pantothenic acid): 500 to 1,000 mg once or twice per day
- Herbs including holy basil (often referred to as tulsi), rhodiola, glycyrrhiza (herbal licorice), and eleutherococcus (Siberian ginseng)

The four herbs listed above are known to increase production of cortisol and potentially adrenaline as well.[2] Glycyrrhiza has been shown to extend the length of time that cortisol is active, which can be an added benefit.[3] You can get these herbs in capsule form, in combinations with nutrients. They also come as herbal tea, tinctures, and even solid extracts (which are like molasses and are taken mixed with water). Note that several of these herbs have been used around the world for centuries. Holy basil is commonly used in India to help with stress. Glycyrrhiza and eleutherococcus are often used in Chinese medicine. Now you can use them to address your stress type.

The timing of your doses is important when it comes to using herbs and nutrients to support cortisol production. Our goal is to reestablish a healthy cortisol curve, where cortisol is higher in the morning and gradually decreasing through the day. You'll want to take your herbal and nutrient support at the time, or just prior to when, your cortisol levels are too low. I think of it like a pothole in the road that we are aiming to fill in, but not overfill, so that as you move through that part of the day, you don't experience a dip in your cortisol levels. You may find you need to take your adrenal/cortisol support in the morning, upon waking, if your levels are low then, and again a couple hours later, around noon and before 3 PM, if your levels dip midday. It's not recommended to support cortisol production after 3 PM because that is when your cortisol naturally decreases.

It's important to be mindful when taking glycyrrhiza. If you have high blood pressure, don't take it until you have managed your blood pressure, because it can raise blood pressure that is already high. It won't cause high blood pressure if your levels are normal. In fact, usually if you have low cortisol and adrenaline, you are likely to have low blood pressure, in which case glycyrrhiza can be very helpful. It is also important to be careful with the quantity of glycyrrhiza. Too high of a dose for too long can cause issues such as muscle breakdown, so don't push your dose too high. Stay at about 250 to 500 mg once or twice per day (before 3 PM).

Some practitioners give almost everyone glandular adrenal support, which contains cortisol, from the get-go, but I find this to be overkill. It could even damage your body by preventing your adrenal glands from recovering. When you take cortisol (or any other hormone) at high doses, it will inhibit the production and function of your own body. Taking cortisol, even in an over-the-counter product, could suppress the ability of your adrenal glands to make cortisol. And your goal here is to help your adrenal glands and body recover from stress, not just to ingest substances that will take over for your adrenals.

Now, again, in some cases, if your adrenal glands are maxed out and simply unable to make more cortisol and adrenaline than they are already making, then glandular support may be necessary, especially as a starting point. Taking the minimum dose, along with herbs and nutrients, can actually give your adrenals a break to recover function. It may take a few months, but what I've found with patients is that with diligent self-care, and just the right amount of filling in for their adrenal glands, they will most often begin to produce cortisol again on their own, even sometimes in cases of Addison's disease and definitely for severe cases of Blah and Blue. Most cases—I would say more than 90 percent—do *not* require hydrocortisone or adrenal glandular cortisol replacement. I don't recommend adding it unless you've already tried the preceding approaches and found that you need more support.

## Support Adrenaline Production if Too Low

If you have low adrenaline levels, such as Sluggish and Stressed, and Blah and Blue, Phase 2 is the time to support adrenaline levels. We can use the precursor nutrient, tyrosine, which is an amino acid. Tyrosine turns into PEA (requires iron), which turns into dopamine, and it converts to norepinephrine and epinephrine (adrenaline). By taking tyrosine, you'll feed into that pathway, supporting dopamine as well. But there is no reason to overdo it. While it is tempting to boost your adrenaline and get some energy, it won't help to go too fast and raise your adrenaline too high. Instead, your goal here is to support your adrenal glands to make just enough adrenaline to keep up with your day.

Note that if you have iron deficiency, which is quite common, your body won't be able to effectively turn tyrosine into adrenaline. Be sure to check your ferritin levels in your blood, and if lower than 50, you'll need to support your iron levels prior to taking tyrosine. I often see this situation arise in women who are experiencing heavy menstrual periods. While one might think our bodies would bleed less when depleted, it is actually the opposite. When iron levels are low, we bleed more, losing still more iron, and lowering adrenaline and energy at the same time.

A common dosage of tyrosine (N-acetyl L-tyrosine) is 25 to 300 mg. Start with a low dose and take it in the morning. It doesn't have to be with food, but I generally suggest taking it with food or a protein shake to avoid nausea that sometimes occurs from swallowing any pill on an empty stomach. Notice how you feel. Does your energy, mood, and motivation level improve? Listen to your body and adjust your doses accordingly. As your adrenal glands recover and your digestion heals, your levels will catch up to optimal, and then you'll likely be able to maintain healthy adrenaline levels without having to take tyrosine every day.

## Balance Your Hormones

It's important at this stage to ensure that you are optimizing your hormones, including thyroid, insulin, estrogen, progesterone, testosterone, and melatonin. I suggest working with a practitioner who has a breadth of experience with optimizing endogenous (from inside your body) hormone production. There is no reason to completely take over your hormone production (or to take it over more than is necessary) if there is a possibility that you can support your body to recover from stress and make adequate hormone levels with the support of natural approaches. In fact, each gland and hormone can be supported with specific nutrients, herbs, and peptides. Helping patients balance hormones (and neurotransmitters) by helping their bodies recover from stress is one of the most rewarding things I do.

## Rebalance Gut Bacteria

An abundance of research has shown that having good gut bacteria benefits our health, while many other studies have indicated that ongoing stress disrupts the balance of our gut bacteria.[4] These discoveries have inspired further research over the past twenty years to figure out how to get our gut bacteria back to where we want them to be. Patients and practitioners have tried flooding the gut with "probiotics," which are mainly composed of two types of bacteria, *Lactobacillus* and *Bifidobacterium*. While taking a probiotic is beneficial to some degree,[5] it is not the "fix-all" everyone hoped for. The reason is that our microbiome is made up of trillions of bacteria, and most do not come in the form of a capsule or powder. Swallowing hundreds of billions of lactobacilli is unlikely to support a diversity of bacteria, which is what we want. Eating a ton of fermented foods is also not going to hit the mark.

Then practitioners started experimenting with fecal transplants that replace one person's microbiome with that of another. But there are risks here, too. We don't want to transfer any unwanted bacteria or infections, and it can be difficult to find the perfect match for what a person lacks. Fecal transplants have been approved in the United States for helping patients with bacteria called *Clostridium difficile* (*C. diff*) because these bacteria are often resistant to antibiotics and patients struggle to get resolution (although I've successfully addressed this condition without antibiotics or fecal transplants). Studies show that fecal transplants have given these patients relief and stopped *C. diff* from causing further issues.[6] Still, these patients need to rebalance their newly transplanted bacteria because the transplant often leaves them in a state of overgrowth, combined with leaky gut that remains from the *C. diff* infection. So fecal transplants are not a perfect solution for everyone, either.

In most cases, the goal is neither to attempt to replace your entire microbiome nor to flood your intestines with a couple of strains. Instead, I suggest first rebalancing your gut bacteria using diet changes, digestive support, stress recovery, and an herbal protocol if needed. Then, once your gut bacteria are optimized, use a probiotic product at a dosage shown to maintain optimal levels over time and during stress exposure.

When it comes down to it, the bacteria and other organisms that live and thrive in our intestines are determined by what we eat and the health of our digestive tract.[7] As you learned in chapter six, eating foods and fiber to feed the bacteria we do want, in quantities that we can digest, combined with strategies to heal leaky gut, is essential for reversing the imbalanced gut bacteria caused by stress. It's also important that your bowels are moving daily because when stool sits in the intestines, that can also cause an overgrowth of bacteria.

If a moderate to severe imbalance of bacteria and/or other organisms exists, then we can use an effective protocol of antimicrobial herbs to address the imbalance or overgrowth. Additionally, rather than using a standard probiotic at this point, I suggest a product containing *Bacillus*, which acts as a kind of traffic director by supporting healthy bacteria and discouraging those we don't want. It is important to begin with low dosages and increase gradually depending on the severity of leaky gut and imbalanced gut bacteria (dysbiosis) in order to prevent an aggravation of symptoms. I am also cautious about using fiber and prebiotics at this point because I don't want to overfeed the bacteria. Arabinogalactan (from the larch plant) is a type of fiber/prebiotic that doesn't overfeed the bacteria and yet helps by supporting health immune function in the intestines.

Another approach, which is considered experimental at this point in time, is helminthic therapy. Studies have demonstrated that, in addition to bacteria, there are other microbes that ought to exist in the human microbiome in order to provide optimal signaling to our digestion, immune system, and nervous system. When these microbes are missing, which is common in developed countries where people are not exposed to them, we have an increased rate of allergies, autoimmunity, and neurological conditions.[8] When very specific microbes are introduced into the intestines, they are able to shift the population of bacteria in a positive way, as well as assist with healing leaky gut, and recalibrate the immune system and nervous system in such a way that the body is essentially reset from stress exposure.[9]

Helminthic therapy has been demonstrated to turn off autoimmunity, without causing negative side effects, which is unheard of for patients otherwise having to take medications with severe side effects. Celiac disease, Crohn's disease, rheumatoid arthritis, and multiple sclerosis have all been helped, amongst many other autoimmune and allergic conditions.[10] And yet helminthic therapy has yet to be used on a large scale. One of the factors that gets in the way is the hygiene hypothesis, which taught that we should be afraid of "germs" and "worms" in particular. While there are certainly parasites that are harmful to humans, just as there are bacteria that are pathogenic, there are also helminths, such as a very specific type of hookworm researchers have identified, that are beneficial to humans. In fact, some argue that humans evolved with hookworms in our bodies, and without them, we are at a disadvantage. I've experienced improvements in my health with hookworm therapy and I've observed its substantial benefit for my patients.

Overall, I want you to know that it is possible to get your gut bacteria back on track with diligence and patience. Patients have proven it to me! Then, once your microbiome is optimized, it is all about keeping it that way. At this point, high-quality probiotics in a supplement form, either capsules or powder, can be helpful. When you purchase a probiotic, you'll want to look for a product that contains multiple strains of two bacteria types: *Lactobacillus* and *Bifidobacterium*. These bacteria are grown by fermentation in labs and were originally used in fermented dairy products (such as yogurt).

Now these bacteria are sold by many different companies in refrigerated and nonrefrigerated forms, and with various quantities and levels of quality of bacteria. When choosing a probiotic product, it is important to know how careful the company was when producing it; this ensures efficacy. Some products are dairy-free, others are free of specific *Lactobacillus* that could trigger histamine reactions for those with that susceptibility. A common maintenance dosage is 25 to 50 billion CFUs (colony-forming units) per day.

## Foundational Nutrients

Certain nutrients are particularly important for helping us recover from and become resilient to stress. These include antioxidants, which we need to counteract oxidative stress, as well as nutrients to decrease inflammation and to support mitochondria. It's important to work with a practitioner who can help you run tests to determine what is depleted or out of balance in your body. Sometimes I imagine this process as a pilot sitting in a cockpit with a hundred dials and gauges. You and your practitioner need to first know what is out of sync (through testing) and then take steps to provide nutrients, or precursor nutrients, so your body can resync all the levels. It's not a quick fix or crutch. It's about choosing nutrients intentionally based on what your body needs to function well.

### Multivitamin and B Vitamins

First, select a multivitamin. Studies show that simply taking a good-quality multivitamin can stave off effects of stress and health conditions, including fatigue, brain fog, and even cancer. A multivitamin will generally contain the basic antioxidants (beta-carotene, vitamins C and E, zinc, and selenium), plus fat-soluble vitamins (E, D, and K), B vitamins (B1, B2, B3, B5, B6, B9, and B12), and additional minerals (such as chromium, manganese, and possibly calcium and magnesium). Some multivitamins contain iron, but that is appropriate only for those who have low iron levels and women who are pregnant, postpartum, and/or breastfeeding.

Too often, however, patients come in with a giant bottle of tablets they purchased at a bargain price. When it comes to vitamins, a bargain price means the manufacturer used cheaper, inactive forms of the nutrients. It doesn't make sense to spend less on vitamins that your body can't use well, especially when high-quality products containing the active form of nutrients don't cost that much more.

By knowing your genetics related to nutrient metabolism, as well as your nutrient levels in blood tests, in particular an intracellular blood test, you and your practitioner can determine whether you have an increased need for certain nutrients. For example, those of us with one or more *MTHFR* gene variations (up to 50 percent of the population) are potentially 30 to 80 percent less able to activate folic acid (the inexpensive, inactive form) into folate (also known as L-methylfolate or 5-MTHF). A homocysteine level on a blood test will tell you if you need more methylfolate, as well as methylcobalamin (B12) and pyridoxine (B6), all of which are involved in the metabolism of homocysteine. Homocysteine above 7 or 8 on the test indicates a need for more folate, B12, and B6.

Working with a naturopathic doctor or clinical nutritionist who specializes in nutrigenomics is extremely helpful for determining the nutrients you need that are specific to your genetics and your history of stress exposure. In the meantime, start with a multivitamin that meets quality standards, is third-party tested, is preferably in capsule form instead of tablets (which are harder to digest), and is free of common allergens and artificial colors. As with anything new that you take, monitor how you feel. If you have any sort of reaction, stop taking the product and consult your practitioner.

It's common to notice that your urine is more yellow when taking a multivitamin or B complex. Once the nutrients are absorbed from your digestion, they travel through your bloodstream to be delivered to your cells. When your blood is filtered by your kidneys, certain nutrients or nutrient metabolites will go into your urine, making it yellow. While many people assume yellow urine means they are "peeing out" their vitamins, in actuality, yellow urine means your body successfully absorbed the nutrients. Having the nutrients come through your bladder in your urine protects your bladder from toxins that may be in your urine as well.

## Omega-3 Fats

Omega-3 fats are also essential for humans, particularly for stress resiliency.[11] We access omega-3s from fish, or fish oil, especially from sardines, mackerel, and salmon. Algae is a vegan source. Some people are able to make omega-3 from omega-6 fats (found in chia seeds and flaxseeds). However, many people (like me) have genetic variations in their metabolism that prevent this conversion. There are two primary types of omega-3 fats—eicosapentaenoic acid (EPA) and docosahexaenoic acid (DHA). Throughout our bodies, they make up the walls of our cells, including nerve cells. To have a healthy body, we need to have healthy cells with cell walls that contain plenty of omega-3 fats. Omega-3 fats also lead down a metabolic pathway that makes substances that counteract inflammation.

Omega-3s have been shown to decrease inflammation, decrease cholesterol, and prevent blood clots. This means that you should be careful taking them if you are on blood thinners or are about to have surgery. Omega-3s have been used to help recovery after traumatic brain injury and stroke; to prevent heart disease in general; to help with skin issues including eczema and acne; to help with joint pain and pain in general; and to help with dementia, anxiety, depression, ADHD, and autoimmune conditions.

Because omega-3 is so helpful in so many ways, and because so many of us aren't getting enough through our diet, I include it in the list of foundational nutrients. A common dosage is 1,000 mg per day (of combined EPA and DHA). Doses of 2,000 to 4,000 mg per day are used clinically for specific conditions. While you can get omega-3s from fish, it's important to be careful about fish consumption as many fish are exposed to metals and toxins. Eating wild salmon, mackerel, and sardines on a regular basis is a good way to get omega-3s through food.

## Magnesium

As I've mentioned, magnesium is one of the most important nutrients for our bodies. It is used in over three hundred biochemical pathways, including the breakdown of adrenaline. Without enough of it, we will be more likely to experience fatigue, anxiety, high blood pressure, muscle cramps, uterine cramps, heart palpitations, headaches, and numbness. At the same time, many of us are deficient in magnesium, especially those who drink alcohol and/or take medications that deplete it (some diuretics, proton pump inhibitors, and antibiotics). We get magnesium in our diet from nuts, seeds, beans, brown rice, oatmeal, white potatoes, spinach, salmon, poultry, beef . . . and chocolate! It's important to choose the type of magnesium based on the desired purpose. Magnesium glycinate is perfect for releasing stress from muscles and the nervous system. A common dose is 100 to 400 mg per day.

## Vitamin D

Vitamin D comes from exposure to sunlight. To be more specific, when our skin is exposed to sunlight, it stimulates the metabolic process of turning cholesterol into vitamin D. This process requires not just any light but specifically ultraviolet B (UVB) light from the sun. Although many of us lack adequate sun exposure, due to not going outdoors or to living at latitudes 37 degrees north or south of the equator during the winter, we can also get vitamin D from certain foods, such as salmon and egg yolk, as well as fortified milk and cereal products.

Vitamin D was first known to be important for helping the intestines absorb calcium and phosphorus, which are important for bone health. Now we know that vitamin D is involved in much more than bones. It supports immune function and decreases inflammation. Vitamin D has been associated with a decreased incidence of heart disease, cancer, and diabetes and a decreased risk of death from any cause. A gene called *VDR* (vitamin D receptor) determines our ability to use vitamin D. If you have variations on this gene, you may require a higher dosage of vitamin D to maintain adequate vitamin D activity.

I recommend having your vitamin D level checked in your blood work at least once per year. The test to order is called 25-OH vitamin D. The optimal level is debated among practitioners, but at this point in time the ideal range is considered to be between 50 and 80 ng/ml. And when you choose a supplement, I suggest taking a daily dose (versus a weekly dose) of 2,000 to 5,000 iu (50 to 1,500 mcg) in a capsule or liquid form of vitamin D3 (not vitamin D2, which is an inactive form). Then recheck your blood levels to determine your best dose.

## Coenzyme Q10

CoQ10 is an important antioxidant to consider. It is a nutrient made inside our bodies, but it is often depleted by stress and oxidative stress. CoQ10 is literally the nutrient used to turn calories to energy in our bodies. Way down deep in our cells, inside the mitochondria, a metabolic and electrical process requiring CoQ10 makes ATP. Without enough of it, we will be lacking in energy. Not only that, but CoQ10 protects our cells from oxidative stress caused by toxin exposure and inflammation.

Every cell in the body uses CoQ10, but one of the most important organs using CoQ10 is the heart. When we are depleted in CoQ10, one of the first symptoms is heart palpitations. This is so much the case that I consider heart palpitations to be a sort of barometer of CoQ10 status in my patients. Once they start taking CoQ10, their heart palpitations often go away, and as they do, I know that all their cells are getting more of this essential nutrient. CoQ10 has been shown to help prevent heart disease, dementia, and migraines and to improve stamina. CoQ10 is depleted as we age, and with the use of statins. CoQ10 is found in meat, fish, and nuts, but the amounts are negligible. Ultimately, we need to consume it in supplement form to keep up with our body's demand. (Note: If you have heart palpitations, it's quite likely that you also need more support for your vagus nerve, as well as magnesium. If you didn't already start taking magnesium based on elevated adrenaline in Phase 1, then it's time to add it. The form of magnesium most beneficial to the heart is magnesium taurate, although threonate and glycinate will also help prevent heart racing and palpitations.)

There has been quite a race in the supplement industry to find a way to make a CoQ10 product that gets absorbed into the body, all the way into the mitochondria. Some people have genetic variations that make it important to take the activated form of CoQ10, called ubiquinol. Finally, a company in New Zealand developed a product called MitoQ that has exceeded all others in terms of delivering CoQ10 to the mitochondria. It has been repeatedly studied and is always identified with more health benefits. This is why I consider MitoQ a foundational supplement. The dosing of MitoQ is different from that of other forms of CoQ10 because absorption is so much better. The dose is 10 to 20 mg per day versus 100 to 400 mg for standard CoQ10 products. My preferred form/brand of CoQ10 is MitoQ because studies show it's the most effective at getting inside cells, to the mitochondria, where it's needed.[12]

### Collagen

Collagen is another important stress resiliency supplement to consider. This supplement is often referred to as collagen peptides and contains amino acids, which makes it a source of protein, although because it does not contain tryptophan, it is considered an "incomplete protein." At the same time, because these amino acids are derived from a food source of collagen (unlike amino acids that are taken individually), they become active once digested and processed in the body. This leads to benefits like improved well-being and decreased risk of disease. Collagen is damaged by, you guessed it, stress! For example, cigarette smoke is a toxin that damages collagen. A diet high in sugar and carbs also damages collagen, as does excessive sun exposure.

When we think about it, we realize that our bodies are largely made up of collagen. Our skin, nails, hair, joints, muscles, tendons, blood vessels, eyes, and connective tissue are all made up of collagen. Collagen within our bodies is made from vitamin C, proline, glycine, and copper. We can access collagen in our diet by consuming bone broth, seafood, poultry, and meats. For a while, scientists wondered if it was possible for collagen that we swallow to turn into collagen within our body structures. Sure enough, studies have confirmed it.[13] This is one reason that taking collagen as a powder or in a capsule has become so popular. It's also because collagen essentially helps us turn back time by reducing wrinkles, improving joint health, increasing muscle strength, healing leaky gut, and preventing bone loss.

A common daily dosage of collagen peptides is between 2.5 and 15 grams. That dose is considered safe and will not disrupt the balance of amino acids in the body. There are at least sixteen different types of collagen in our bodies, but 90 percent of it is types I, II, and III, so a product that is mainly made up of these types of collagen is preferable. You can find collagen products that are marine derived (from fish) or bovine derived (from cows). When choosing marine collagen, make sure the label says "wild caught." For bovine collagen, be sure the label indicates that the animals were grass fed.

## Balancing Protein Shake

I like to start my day with a protein shake. I do this for several reasons. First, starting with protein means that my blood sugar levels will be managed. Second, it means that I get adequate protein for energy and muscle support. I add my leaky gut healing powder (with glutamine, DGL, aloe, and arabinogalactan fiber), flaxseed oil, liquid berry extract, and collagen powder to my protein shake, which makes it an easy way for me to get in healthy fats, phytonutrients, and gut healing. I mix my shake in water to avoid adding extra calories and carbs, and as I'm swallowing my protein shake, I swallow my foundational supplements and Stress Recovery Protocol supplements along with it. In this way, I'm efficiently giving my body what it needs to be as resilient as possible to stress throughout the day.

Note that I don't add a whole bunch of fruit and greens to my shake because the fruit can add carbs and the greens can add more oxalates than I need. I choose a protein powder that does not contain added sugar; there's no reason to put sugar in this when I'm having the shake to be healthy! I prefer to use an organic pea protein powder because it tastes good, is dairy-free (versus one that uses whey protein, a common food allergen), and doesn't contain arsenic (some rice protein powders do contain arsenic).

Instead of, or in addition to, having a protein shake in the morning, you may find it works better for you to have a shake at midday or in the evening, to replace a carb-filled meal or snack. If you prefer sweetness, you can sweeten your shake with stevia or monk fruit instead of sugar. Choosing a protein powder that is flavored with vanilla or chocolate can make your shake taste like a treat, even though it is good for you. You could add avocado or nut butter and blend to make your shake creamier. Add cinnamon to make it more like a spiced drink. Add ice and blend to make it like a smoothie. I've even had patients who freeze their protein shakes to make them into frozen desserts. Find a couple of my favorite recipes using protein powder in the recipe section of this book.

## RECOMMENDED SUPPLEMENTS AND SHAKES

If you're looking for a reliable source for your supplements, including many of those I've mentioned in chapters ten and eleven, I recommend my product line, Nature Empowered Nutritionals. Visit DoctorDoni. com to find them.

## Creating a Support Network

As you support the networks within your body, it is the perfect time to set up support around you in terms of human connections. Studies show that developing a social network improves health.[14]

Be you, without the old masks and ways of being that were only adding to your stress. Communicate with your loved ones and let them know about the work you are doing to master your stress and reset your health. Share with them your feelings of gratitude for their support, let them know what you need, and find out how you can be a support to them as your health improves.

It is also important to consider the relationships in your life: Do they provide you with love and opportunities for emotional growth, or are they filled with stress and negativity? If you feel that you need new forms of community and connection, take time to meditate and/or journal about how that would look and feel to you. As you participate in stress recovery activities or take on new hobbies, look for opportunities to join in-person and/or online communities of people who are also focused on self-growth and mastery.

Use the spiritual elements to guide you and remind you that strength within comes with support around you. You are not alone. We are all in this world and life together (earth). As you communicate your authentic feelings and values, you are essentially stepping into the fire and giving others permission to do the same (fire). We can then flow through life as water flows, cleansing and nurturing us (water). We all require air, which we breathe in and out, to receive much needed oxygen and renewal (air). Reminding ourselves of our interconnectedness helps release stress and allows our adrenals and stress response system to repair.

## Phases of Recovery for Your Stress Type

### Stress Magnet

In Phase 2, you may find that you need to support your adrenal gland function with nutrients and herbs, but only if your levels have decreased and are below optimal. Otherwise, during Phase 2 you may be continuing to monitor and prevent cortisol and adrenaline from rising again. You may also use Phase 2 to start working to rebalance other hormones that have been disrupted by stress, such as thyroid hormones, insulin, ovarian or testicular hormones, and so on. You'll also want to work on healing your digestion. Now that your cortisol (and adrenaline) is out of stress mode, they will actually help to rebalance other systems in your body and maintain a healthier state.

## Night Owl

In Phase 2, you may need to address cortisol levels that are too low in the morning. This is not always the case, but if you've been in the Night Owl pattern for a rather long time, your adrenals may actually be completely lopsided from making cortisol at night instead of in the morning. Once you've calmed your system and decreased cortisol and adrenaline at night, you'll be ready to increase cortisol and adrenaline in the morning. Go slowly, so as not to shift things too quickly. Your body will guide you. Little by little, you'll be able to reteach your body how to have a morning cortisol response and how to make cortisol trend downward in the evening.

## Sluggish and Stressed

When you get to Phase 2, you'll be ready to start supporting adrenaline production with tyrosine and perhaps other nutrients and herbs to help your adrenal glands recover. It's tricky because you want to support the production of adrenaline, but you don't want to increase cortisol too high and swing right back into stress mode. So just go carefully, use tyrosine without herbs, and notice if symptoms return; if they do, you can adjust doses accordingly.

## Blah and Blue

Your cortisol is too low in the morning, so take herbs such as rhodiola, holy basil, and glycyrrhiza, along with vitamin B5 and vitamin C, to help kick-start the production of cortisol and adrenaline by your adrenal glands. You should take it slowly because, ironically, when your body is used to functioning with low cortisol and adrenaline, it can feel overstimulating to increase them. I find that many people feel that "slowly but surely" is better than a fast acceleration. Start with low doses, of one or more ingredients, and allow your body to guide you to increase or repeat the doses in the morning and at midday until you find what best fits you, for now. As your adrenals recover, doses may change or decrease, but the key is that you should absolutely feel some change. If you don't feel any difference at all, you need to change products or consider adding cortisol support in the form of a glandular product or low dose of hydrocortisone for a period of time.

For adrenaline support, add in tyrosine, again, starting at low doses so as not to jolt your system. You may need to take tyrosine in the morning and at midday. And if you have a *COMT* gene variation, you are likely to need less tyrosine to make a difference. If ever you feel that you supported your adrenaline too much, then take some magnesium threonate to correct the issue by helping to support COMT. Within a few tweaks, you'll find the best dose and timing for you.

Keep in mind that the support for cortisol and adrenaline is having an immediate effect, but it is also giving you a long-term benefit by helping your adrenals recover. This is not a crutch or mask. This approach is helping your adrenal glands improve their function, and they will be able to maintain that benefit for as long as you continue to implement self-care and provide appropriate nutrient and herbal support for your body. I say this from many years of personal experience. I tend toward the Blah and Blue type myself and found myself in full stress mode about fifteen years ago. I've since been able to prevent that situation by staying ahead of the curve.

## Tired and Wired

As adrenaline decreases, you'll add in adrenal support in order to increase cortisol; just be careful so as not to raise your adrenaline all over again. In fact, you may want to start with a product that doesn't contain tyrosine and focus on vitamin C, B vitamins, and gentle restorative herbs like holy basil. As your system stabilizes, you'll be able to add in stronger herbs, like rhodiola and glycyrrhiza, to raise your cortisol. These herbs can also increase adrenaline, so go slowly, and stop or add in more magnesium if you feel your adrenaline rise too high again.

# Phase 3 | Resilience

I t's time to become a pro at being resilient to stress.

You've worked hard through Phases 1 and 2 to help your body and adrenal glands recover from stress exposure. Now I want to help you keep things that way. You should be proud of what you've achieved. The last thing we want to see is a return to stress mode.

At the same time, you are human, and humans are not perfect! Plus, as you start to feel better, it's tempting to do more and push the limits a bit more.

If you fall right back into your usual stress exposure, at work, at home, in relationships, and in life in general, it's quite possible that you will slide back into stress mode. If you do slide back into that realm, try not to be hard on yourself, and take solace in the fact that you now know what is happening and what to do about it.

It's quite likely that you'll catch imbalances earlier this time, before they become severe. When you've been feeling good, it is a lot easier to notice if something doesn't feel well. And if you've been establishing a self-care routine along the way, you'll know just what to implement to get yourself back on track.

I find that patients are often so relieved to feel better that they are more motivated than ever to find ways to maintain this state and re-create their life in a way that accommodates how they now feel. At this point, it's all about time management as you more intentionally choose optimal stresses for your body, creating a routine for self-care, and making the most of the tools in the previous chapters by integrating them effectively into your schedule.

Maintenance is about creating systems that help you remain de-stressed and balanced over time—systems sustainable specifically for your lifestyle. For instance, with eating habits, one reader might need to prep food for the week every Sunday, while another might hire a delivery service to bring food to their door every day. These systems or routines become like a safety net to keep you on track with C.A.R.E. even as you choose to explore more opportunities in your environment or in the world.

That's why I use the term *resiliency*, which means the ability to recover from difficult conditions quickly. A resilient object is able to spring back into shape after being bent or compressed. That is what I envision for you: the ability to bounce back from any stress that comes along and return your body to optimal cortisol and adrenaline levels, and back to balanced hormones and neurotransmitters and functioning digestive and immune systems. It's not about expecting that you can avoid all difficulties. Instead, it is about accepting that you are human and you'll experience stress, and being ready with stress recovery tools and techniques that allow you to be you and experience even more of what you'd like to experience in your life.

Stress doesn't go away entirely. Truthfully, we can't escape it. I don't encourage you to try to avoid all stress, because the more you try to escape stress, the more you will stress yourself out trying. In fact, as you feel better, you'll want to choose challenges and projects that bring you joy and fulfill your purpose. The goal is to create a stress support system that will prevent you from reverting to burnout mode. That stress support system includes vitamins and supplements that have been shown to help maintain resilience to stress. A life that includes both stress and stress recovery becomes your new, enjoyable normal because you're taking care of yourself and filling your time with things that nurture who you are and what you want to do most—without the burden of adrenal distress.

## Defining and Maintaining Resilience

Living in Phase 3 is the goal.

Here cortisol is highest in the morning, but not too high, and decreases gradually throughout the day, until it is lowest while you sleep at night. Adrenaline is produced and metabolized at a steady level, giving you the energy to do what you want and need to do, but not so much or so little that it will cause waves in your day.

I think of stress recovery as a boat on a lake. (I grew up boating every summer, so I'm very familiar with the feel of being on a boat under calm and rough conditions.) When the waters are calm, you feel a gentle rock, and things balance back out easily. When you hit a wake, it can feel like a jolt. You brace yourself. It may take a bit longer to recover, but soon enough you feel back in balance again, gliding across the water smoothly. When the waters are rough and the waves are rolling in one after the next, it is hard to know what is up and what is down, or when the storm is going to stop. You lose track of center, and that's what causes seasickness (been there, done that!). You can't wait to get back to the dock, and once you do, it takes time for your body to know that it's off the waves and back onshore. Recovering from stress is quite like this.

It can take time, but we can signal to our bodies that we're back onshore. Then we can recover from stress while continuing to navigate the waves that will come next time we head out on the water.

Resiliency is not masking a superficial deficiency, nor is it about getting off the roller coaster of life altogether. It requires that you first complete Phases 1 and 2 to create internal balance and a point of reference that is centered. Then you are ready to master the ability to choose your optimal stress and to support yourself based on your body's patterns. It takes practice. You'll get good at knowing how much of which stress is good for you, and when too much pushes you over your stress threshold. You'll be able to take on projects, live your purpose, and excel, without going overboard and knocking yourself out.

## Routines Matter

Routine is the language our bodies speak. In fact, our bodies are actually de-stressed by having routines. We live on the planet Earth, which circles the sun every 365 days. Furthermore, this Earth of ours rotates the sun every twenty-four hours, creating day and night.

Our brains respond to these built-in environmental routines. They signal our hormone production, immune function, and ability to access nutrients through our skin, our food, and the nutrients made by the bacteria living in our intestines. Even the moon that orbits around Earth every twenty-seven days affects our bodies, influencing when our ovaries ovulate and how much melatonin is produced. The more we distance ourselves from these environmental signals by, for example, exposing ourselves to light at night or not spending time in nature, the more of a stress this is to our bodies, and the more the healthy signaling goes awry.

One of the best ways to give our bodies their best chance at being resilient to stress is by providing a foundational schedule, so our bodies don't have to constantly adapt to our environment. By creating a relative constant, we ensure that any other variables that come along—say, being woken in the night by a child or having a deadline at work—can be handled with ease, as we return to our usual routines. By purposely creating a routine of wake time and sleep time, time for work, time to relax, time for movement, and time for eating, we are giving our bodies signals they can count on and relate to.

There may be times when you need to change your routine, like when you travel or during a pandemic, in which case you can make changes with intention and prioritize regularity as efficiently as you can. This will help you adapt to the stress at hand.

At the same time, I don't believe there is one routine that is best for everyone. Genetics, personality, preferences, and stress type come into play when creating a routine. So I encourage you to take into account your uniqueness and use this as a chance to know yourself better and give yourself what you need. If someone or something else has been determining your routine for quite a long time, it may seem foreign to create it with intention. Be patient with yourself and use journaling and meditation to guide you. And listen to the signals your body gives you in terms of energy, sleep, mood, focus, and other symptoms to let you know whether your routine is working for you. Now, let's take a look at the factors to consider when assessing your routine, including chronotype.

## CLOCK Genes Unpacked

We talked about circadian rhythm in chapter seven when talking about sleep. Our sleep-wake cycle is very much (50 percent) determined by genes referred to as CLOCK genes. These genes influence when we each tend to go to sleep and wake up, despite stress, work, and everything else going on in our lives. These tendencies are called chronotypes.

If you tend to stay up late, which is more common for teens, you have a late chronotype. If you tend to wake up early, as tends to happen for children and people over sixty, you have an early chronotype. Most of us fall in the middle. As you get out of stress mode, the effect your chronotype is having on your sleep schedule will become more apparent.

I often joke with my friends that I live on West Coast time, because I lived on the West Coast for thirty years of my life. Even though I've lived on East Coast time for twenty years now, I still tend to go to sleep around midnight. And that is with low cortisol and adrenaline at night, so I'm not in Night Owl stress mode. That is my body's chronotype. When I asked my mom, she confirmed that I tended to stay up late as a child. And my daughter has this same chronotype, so it seems I passed my CLOCK genes on to her.

Knowing your chronotype can be helpful because it allows you to plan your day based on your best sleep-wake cycle. If you plan on an early-morning workout and you do not have an early chronotype, you are likely going to feel exhausted and give up on the exercise routine because it simply doesn't match up with your body. Being able to plan your self-care, as well as your work and other necessary tasks, based on your optimal times of day can be life changing in terms of improving your efficiency and the way you feel.

## Reset Your Personal Autopilot

Much of what we do each day is on autopilot.

Imagine if you had to think through every single task you do each day, from brushing your teeth to driving your car, as if you were doing that task for the first time. It would be totally exhausting! Instead, a part of our brain called the basal ganglia is able to automate some things that we do repeatedly. When you want to integrate new activities into your routine, it's going to take some time and repetition for your basal ganglia to get them set up and auto-mated. During this time, a bit of effort will be required on your part.

One trick I use when adding a new habit to my routine is to tell myself to do it around the time that I already do something else that I know is on auto. For example, when I wanted to start taking vitamin C for my teeth and immune system, as well as my nervous system and glutathione recycling system, I decided I'd take it right after I brush my teeth each night. I know I'm going to brush my teeth. That is a well-established pattern. All I had to do was think, "Brush teeth, take vitamin C." And after doing it a few times, it stuck. I mention this trick to patients when they are trying to get into the routine of taking a new supplement or remember to bring a protein snack when leaving the house. Tie the new habit to an old habit and, voilà, you'll remember.

Our brains respond much better to positive associations, too. What this means is that when we give ourselves a reward, we are more likely to choose that behavior in the future. It is like training a dog. When you give the dog a treat, it is more likely to sit or heel. Same for us humans. This is referred to by neuroscientists as a cue-response-reward cycle. An example would be eating chocolate or doing something enjoyable after studying or finishing a project.

It can seem too simple to make things easy for yourself, but, hey, when you know that's how your brain works best, you might as well give it what it needs to achieve the best results. When you want to create a new routine or habit for yourself, think about it in terms of what you can do immediately afterward that will give your brain a signal that you enjoy this new habit. This will allow you to establish your new routine more easily and much faster.

I also want to acknowledge that some of us prefer to integrate variety into our routines. If following the same routine and doing the same activities seems boring to you, you are likely a person who needs to mix it up a bit. It's possible to create variety while still making sure that your body gets the benefit of a regular routine and you get adequate self-care time. Try choosing different types of exercise each day, and try scrambling the order in which you imple-ment your preferred stress-reducing activities. For example, some days I wake up and meditate first thing, then walk outside or take a swim, before taking a shower and having a protein shake. Other days I go straight into a low-impact strength workout or Pilates, and then take time to listen to a mindfulness or guided imagery session later in the day.

One thing to definitely include in your routine is breaks. They can be short breaks (or long breaks if needed). Even one minute every hour can make a difference. Studies show that when we take breaks, our stress level decreases and our creativity and productivity increase.[1] In the moment it can seem like you don't have time to take a break, but in actuality, taking a break will help you accomplish more in the long run.

Don't feel that you have to do the exact same thing, in the exact same way, at the exact same time every day. That might just create more stress! What's more important is that you are consistent in when you wake, when you go to sleep, and the intervals of time between meals, and that you regularly take breaks, spend time in nature, and participate in stress recovery activities.

## Create a Healthful Schedule

To take back your health requires intention and a plan. You may need to write your new schedule down, put it into your calendar, and tell those around you that this is your new agenda. It may help to let them know that you realized you need to put C.A.R.E. into your schedule for it to happen, and that you might not be available at the same times they are used to having access to you. You may want to share that you're taking steps to improve your health, and that you're learning as you go, so your schedule may shift until you find the best way of being.

Start by thinking through your day and week. What are your usual work hours? Is this schedule working for you, or does it need to shift a bit? What are your best sleep hours? Set these hours in your schedule. Is there anything else you need to do on a regular basis? A class you go to, a church or temple service you attend, a care routine you have for your parents, volunteer work you do, an activity you bring your children to, or an event or meeting you regularly attend? Put those into the schedule, too.

Keep in mind that anything in your schedule can move. Nothing is set in stone. If you need something to shift, there is a way. It may require a conversation that you've been avoiding or a decision you haven't wanted to make. It could also mean that you need more help getting tasks done or caring for your children, pets, home, or parents than you have considered in the past. But there's only so much you can do in a day. You need to figure out what you are doing now that might be able to be dropped out or delegated. To start, make a list of possibilities. Don't feel that you are committing to anything at this moment. It's just a brainstorm. What could someone else do for you?

Delegating is a process of identifying what you do best, including which activities absolutely need to be done by you and which activities could be done by someone else. In a business, there are processes and tasks that need to be done repeatedly. Each process has a set of steps, takes a certain amount of time, and could be "batched" so the same steps are repeated in a block of time to improve efficiency. The same can be done for your home care. Doing the laundry, for example, is a process that needs to be repeated. When done in a batch, it's completed most efficiently. The same goes for cleaning the house, opening mail, shopping for food and cooking it, doing the dishes, making the bed, and getting ready for bed.

It may help to closely examine a few days and write down everything that you do each day. What is the best time of day and frequency for each task? What are the steps involved? How long does it take? Is this something that only you can do, or could another person do it for you? Better yet, could it be automated?

You can also add up the amounts of time that you spend on your most essential tasks to get a total for the day, and the week. Then subtract that number from the total amount of time in a day and week, and then subtract the number of hours that you need to sleep. This will give you the amount of extra time you have available for other self-care activities.

What do you notice? Do you have the right amount of time for self-care? Too little? Too much (this is less common, but it does happen, and can be stressful, as well)?

I remember when I first went through this process and started to think of each task and activity with intention. It was at a point in my life when I was completely overwhelmed and felt that I never had a minute to myself without feeling exhausted or having a migraine. I realized that I had to get ahead of it. If I didn't intentionally start making changes and decisions, it would keep on happening the same way, day after day, and I would continue to feel worse and worse. So one day I decided to start making shifts. I didn't change everything overnight, but I did start by identifying one task that someone else could do instead of me. I was a single mom without family living nearby, so I didn't have others in the household to help. I needed to create a line item in my budget for me to hire the best person for that task. Once I was able to afford it and found the right person, we set a schedule for when I could expect that person to do that task for me, and once I handed over the task, I was able to insert my own self-care into that time slot.

I invite you to take a look at how you are spending your time, with the intention of finding time that you can then attribute to self-care. Do this without pressure, expectation, and judgment; they only create more stress. With gentleness and the intention of nurturing, ask yourself, "How do I want to spend time in my life? What do I want to be doing, contributing, and accomplishing? And how do I want to be feeling as I do it?" If not feeling well is taking up too much time, let's change that. Let's create a schedule that allows you to take care of you, first and foremost.

## Monitor Resiliency

Patients sometimes ask me how they will know that what they are doing is working. How will they know that choosing healthier foods, getting more sleep, taking supplements, adding stress recovery activities, and making time for exercise are actually paying off? I get it. They don't want to do something that isn't making a difference, and they want to know that it's worth their while.

Some people can tell right away, simply because they feel better. Patients have reported feeling ten or even fifteen years younger than they are now. They say, "I feel like I did when I was forty," for example.

When your energy, mood, and focus improve, it's easy to notice that you feel like a new you! Sometimes these changes happen gradually, so they are less noticeable. Perhaps others notice before you do and say things like, "Wow, you look great! Did you get a haircut?"

That's the thing: when your bod is more resilient to stress, you'll start looking better, and your hair, skin, and even your posture will appear different from the outside. At the same time, you may find yourself wanting to do things you haven't done in a long time. It gets tempting to do more, take on new tasks and projects, say yes to helping others, and exercise more.

Please be careful, because when you pass your new limit, you are likely to find yourself on the couch for a couple of days recovering again. Now that you've recovered from stress mode, your body is more likely to tell you when you've hit your limit. It can feel frustrating at first. You may find yourself questioning your body as to what happened. And then, with a bit of introspection, you'll likely realize, "Oh yeah, I ate something I haven't eaten in a while, and I stretched myself beyond my limit a few too many times." Your body will remind you if you've done too much, and likely with the same symptoms as those you faced and struggled with in the past (or similar symptoms). Heartburn, a headache, or joint pain will be back to remind you that you overdid it. You are human, after all.

Usually, if my patients go back into stress mode, they fit the same stress type they had in the past. Occasionally it shifts to a different stress type. If you return to stress mode, doing the assessment again will ensure you know how best to help your body recover. In fact, I suggest checking in with yourself on a weekly and quarterly basis to see how you are doing in terms of your energy level and stamina; sleep hours and timing; mental focus and memory; mood; and body symptoms.

If you tend toward high cortisol as a Stress Magnet or Sluggish and Stressed, you'll know to add back in banaba leaf and phosphatidylserine at the time of day that your cortisol is too high. If your cortisol is too low, then you'll want to take adrenal-supportive herbs and nutrients, or increase your doses, to match what your body needs at that point in time to stay in the resiliency zone.

The good news is that once you've recovered from stress, your body has learned how to do that, too, and it will be a lot easier to recover next time. Patients describe feeling better in days to weeks, versus months the first time around. Just know that it is normal to take steps forward in terms of your health, and then a step back every so often. This is part of the learning and recovery process. Expect three steps forward and one step back. As time goes on, this will add up to lots of forward movement. If you have a bad day, or feel worse, keep in mind all that has been going well, what you've learned about what your body needs, and that doing these things will make you feel better again. There's no reason to be hard on yourself; that is just another form of stress.

We need to shift the pattern of how we handle stress in order to prevent adrenal distress from happening again. Some people approach this by "being positive," and there are certainly studies that show that being optimistic makes a difference.[2] For others, this approach seems too superficial, unrealistic, and/or dismissive of authentic feelings.[3]

Instead, let's bring the focus back to giving our bodies (and brains) what they need to be successful and healthy. Anything else is simply working against us. Accept that this is the body you live in. These are your genes, your stress exposure, and your stress type. Now, with that information, what will you do with the body you live in? Do you want to be mad at yourself and create more stress, or forgive yourself for being human and learn from the experience?

You've got this. Studies show that it is possible to create new neural pathways.[4] Our brains and nervous systems are not set in stone. If we change the environment and input into our nervous systems, they can learn new patterns. In fact, this is one of the key benefits of many of the stress recovery activities we discussed in chapter eight. They support the growth of new neural pathways. This is true of mindfulness and meditation. And biofeedback helps establish new neural pathways and can be used to establish positive emotional states plus new routines. Use these tools to help you shift away from stress patterns and toward resiliency.

As you do, you are also using epigenetics to positively affect your gene expression. The genes that turned on and created your stress type can turn off again. The same goes for the genes that predispose you to certain health issues. Just as stresses epigenetically increase your risk of disease, anti-stress epigenetically decreases your risk. You can literally reset your health by mastering your stress.

Heart rate variability (HRV) and heart rate coherence can be used to monitor and evaluate your state of resiliency to stress. Using a device that measures your HRV on a regular basis, you'll be able to have an objective measure, right in front of you, that shows you how what you are doing is making a difference. Remember, when we are in stress mode, HRV decreases.

As you implement C.A.R.E., which includes ways of eating, sleeping, recovering from stress, and exercising, all of which are known to improve HRV, you'll see an increase in your HRV. You'll also find that you achieve a greater balance between sympathetic and parasympathetic systems, which is the definition of resilience. You will be ready to respond to stress when it comes along and as you choose your optimal stress activities, but you will also be just as ready to rest and recover, based on your stress type, once the stress is gone.

## C.A.R.E. in a Daily Routine

Now for the fun part.

Think of the C.A.R.E. information in chapters six through nine as a complete self-care menu for your life. Pick and choose what piqued your interest and inspired you to want to make changes in your routine. What matched up with your stress type in terms of C.A.R.E.? What would you like to try implementing in order to see how it feels and what works for you? It may be different now from what it will be as you progress through the Stress Recovery Protocol, and that is okay. It's important to listen to your intuition when deciding what to try. No matter what you start with, you'll be able to learn and grow and adjust as you go.

First, I'm going to share a sample daily routine with times, so that you can get a sense of how it fits in a twenty-four-hour time frame. Then I'll share sample daily routines for each stress type. I want you to have an example and guide to follow and try out. Pay attention to how you feel and make adjustments as needed.

### Sample Day of C.A.R.E.

As you read through this example day, please keep in mind that it is a sample. Don't feel that you have to fit into this schedule exactly. I'm providing it just to give you a sense of how everything fits in and how a schedule could look for you. Of course, there will be variations based on your life, work, commute, priorities, chronotype, and stress type and where you are in the Stress Recovery Protocol. The idea is for you to get a sense of what to aim for and where to focus on making gradual shifts.

> 7:00 AM: Wake up and meditate for (at least) fifteen minutes (it's okay to go to the bathroom first if needed).
>
> 7:15 AM: Practice gratitude and pray. What are you thankful for? What are your intentions for the day?
>
> 7:30 AM: It's time for the exercise or movement of your choice. Get some sunlight exposure if possible. Walk your dog or take a cold swim if you can.

8:00 AM: Drink a protein shake and take morning supplements. If you feel ready to extend your overnight fast, you can delay your shake for a couple of hours.

8:15 AM: Shower, brush your teeth, and get dressed. Perhaps put on music or a motivating podcast.

8:30 AM: Head to work or your office. Organize your thoughts and prioritize tasks.

9:00 AM: You're ready to work or focus on a project. What would you like to get done today? Are there any phone calls you need to make or tasks you want to get done? Do them now if possible.

10:00 AM: Now and every hour while working, take a break for a few minutes. Go to the bathroom, drink water, stretch or do a few squats, clear your mind, and check in with yourself.

Noon: It's time to eat again in order to maintain healthy blood sugar levels and energy. Perhaps you have a nut-based protein bar or a small lunch containing protein and leafy greens or veggies. Take nice deep breaths before you sit down to eat. Set aside other tasks for the moment and focus on feeding yourself healthy nutrients. Pay attention to each bite as you chew carefully.

1:00, 2:00, and 3:00 PM: Remember to take breaks to use the bathroom, drink water, take a few deep breaths, check your priority list for the day, take a walk, and get perspective on how things are going. Do you need to debrief with a friend or assistant?

3:00 or 4:00 PM: It's time to eat again, perhaps a second lunch, with protein. Are there supplements you need to take at this time to help manage stress mode?

5:00 PM: Optimally, your workday will be done by now or wrapping up. Think about or write down what you accomplished and anything you need to continue tomorrow. Reply to messages and make arrangements for what can be done later. Start to wind down your brain. It may be a good time for a walk outside or a meditation.

6:00 to 7:00 PM: It's dinnertime, so set aside your worries and tasks, and sit down to enjoy another digestible-sized meal containing protein and healthy fats, without inflammatory foods or sugar. Drink a small amount of water or herbal tea; try to avoid carbonated beverages and alcohol. Take supplements and digestive enzymes.

8:00 PM: Talk to whoever may be joining you. Share your thoughts and experiences of the day with a sense of gratitude and pleasure. Read a bedtime story to your kids. Snuggle on the couch with your sweetheart or pet and watch a show you enjoy (not a show that increases adrenaline) and/or have sex. If you're looking for a new relationship, journal about what it will look like and feel like to have a loving partner in your life.

9:00 PM: What do you need to do before bed? Turn off your computer and phone, turn down the lights, perhaps take a bath (with Epsom salts), listen to calming music or the sound of a fire crackling, take your evening supplements, brush your teeth, and wash your face. Apply moisturizer, castor oil (which is anti-inflammatory and antispasmodic and helps move lymph), and/or CBD oil as needed to your skin and achy joints/muscles so these substances can work while you sleep.

10:00 to 10:30 PM: Plan to be heading to bed and ready for affirmations and a meditation or yoga nidra to help you progressively relax and get into sleep mode. Set the temperature where you need it, close the shades, turn out the lights, and turn on any sleep-supportive music or sounds.

10:30 PM to 7:00 AM: Sleep and restore! There is so much you get done while you sleep; remind yourself of this, and celebrate the hours that go by while you are in a slumber.

Does this sound like your life? In what way does it sound familiar? Are there ideas you can take from this that you'd like to integrate into your schedule? What do you think would, or wouldn't, work well for you? Journal about this and make note of what you'd like to try.

As you start to try out changes to your schedule, it is perfectly fine to start with one part of your day—the morning, for example—and then, as you get that figured out, move on to adjusting the middle part of your day. Again, the idea here is to make gradual changes. Be gentle with yourself. If something goes "wrong," it's really a learning opportunity that's letting you know what would work better. Take it at your own pace. You do *not* need to make any overnight, cold-turkey changes. In fact, for some people, making too many changes at once might cause the whole effort to backfire.

Being a parent adds an extra challenge to fitting in time for yourself. I get it. When my daughter was young, she provided many opportunities for me to figure this out. One idea is to include your child or children in the self-care routine whenever possible. These activities are good for children, too, and what better time to learn how to create a self-care schedule than as a child? They can meditate with you or join you on a walk or in an exercise session, and can also benefit from taking breaks, especially when they are doing school from home. I also found that I could sometimes combine activities for my daughter with self-care for me. For example, when I was waiting for her to come out of a dance class, it was the perfect time for me to meditate in the car. While making her lunch, folding laundry, or walking her to the bus or train, I could be practicing gratitude in my mind or listening to music or a podcast that helped me recenter and gain perspective.

For those of you who work or study from home, setting up a schedule for yourself is critical; otherwise, you may find yourself in front of your computer, partway through the day, caught up in the vortex of social media or email messages, before you even have a chance to get dressed, let alone eat food or get centered. Creating a structure and sticking to it will establish boundaries for you and for others in your life, on your work team, or in your classes. You may find that it helps to put your schedule into a shared calendar and to set reminder alerts for yourself, including for your recentering and break times.

Once you have prioritized self-care and have a sense of which activities you enjoy, it will become second nature to choose these activities as you go through your day. And as the people in your life get used to seeing you choose self-care, it will be expected, and they may even join you!

## Routines for Happiness and Health for Your Stress Type

Now let's look at sample C.A.R.E. routines based on your stress type. The idea here is that C.A.R.E. is not a one-size-fits-all plan. While self-care, eating healthy, getting enough sleep, implementing stress recovery, and exercising are good in general for all humans, the specifics of how you integrate C.A.R.E. into your day are unique to you. They're also unique to where you are in the Stress Recovery Protocol.

If you are in Phase 1, getting out of stress mode, then it's particularly important to follow C.A.R.E. based on your stress type. As you get out of stress mode and move on to Phase 2, you may find that your best C.A.R.E. routine shifts a bit. That's a good thing. By the time you get to Phase 3, resiliency, it is all about maintaining your progress and preventing stress mode from happening again. At that point, you'll want to focus on C.A.R.E. that helps you respond and recover from stress, but without causing more stress to your system. It's about finding that perfect balance and about hormesis and homeostasis—you need to provide just enough of a challenge for your body to continue to function and allow you to do what you'd like to do in life, but not so much of a challenge that it throws off your homeostatic balance point. That is resiliency. That is your goal.

Remember to include the spiritual elements of earth, fire, water, and air in your C.A.R.E. routine.

## Stress Magnet

C: Have mini meals on hand to eat every three to four hours throughout the day. Have carbs from veggies, fruit, or gluten-free grains along with protein and healthy fats.

A: Put on blue-light-blocking glasses in the evening. Meditate before bed at or by 10 PM, and when you wake.

R: Take one- to five-minute breaks during the day to take a few deep breaths, meditate, spend time outdoors, or listen to music.

E: Implement five minutes of stretching or yoga, then five to ten minutes of core strengthening.

## Night Owl

C: Eat at regular intervals throughout the day, and then at night choose protein, carbs, and healthy fats to balance blood sugar and hormones.

A: Set aside the evening to dim the lights, listen to calming music, and take a bath, and then pull down the blackout shades and practice progressive relaxation.

R: Spend time in nature, especially in the morning. Take deep breaths, journal, or call a friend.

E: Exercise up to thirty minutes a day, before 3 PM. Do Pilates or go for a walk outside.

## Sluggish and Stressed

C: Reach for a protein shake in the morning, and choose small meals containing a slightly higher amount of carbohydrates than protein and fat throughout the day.

A: Set aside "you time" in the evening to journal, call a friend, or listen to music.

R: When you wake, start with a meditation or mindfulness walk in nature. Take breaks during the day.

E: At midday, aim for strengthening, such as a ten-minute LIIT workout or Pilates.

## Blah and Blue

C: Eat a meal/snack, served on a small plate, every two to four hours. Check to be sure it contains protein and healthy fat to prevent your blood sugar from dropping.

A: Enjoy getting ready for bed. Pamper yourself, wrap yourself in a cozy blanket, and play some healing music.

R: Making time for yourself is a good thing. Draw, paint, sing, play music, dance, color, and laugh.

E: Movement upon waking is a nice choice. Start with gentle stretching or yoga and increase to Pilates or a walk outside.

## Tired and Wired

C: You may want to delay breakfast a bit to do an intermittent fast. Then choose protein with easy-to-digest carbs and healthy fats throughout the day.

A: Decompress in the evening by putting work away and choosing calming activities instead.

R: Get fresh air, take a short walk, notice nature, and practice biofeed-back; it may also help to think of positive feelings as you breathe.

E: Alternate different types of exercise in the morning, starting with ten to fifteen minutes of core strengthening, HIIT, or aerobic exercise such as stairs or an elliptical machine.

# Conclusion

## Change Your Stress POV, Change Your Life

We tend to get used to our schedule the way it is. Next thing we know, we look back over a year, or a decade for that matter, and realize, "Oh my gosh, I've been doing the same thing every day and every week." Getting ready for work, going to work, getting through the workday, eating at the same café, dealing with one deadline after the next, working toward the next holiday or vacation. Meanwhile, our kids get older, and so do our parents and pets. Every so often, we might get a moment to stop and look around at our life, and think, "Am I doing what I love?"

What if we can intentionally put a break into our schedules each month, each week, or even each day? Does your schedule allow you to have a day each week to just sit or do whatever you please? Could you create that? Do you have five minutes in each day when you can be with yourself and quietly reflect on what you are grateful for and what you'd like to attract in your life? Where could that fit in your day? How do you create time for *you*?

Learn from the moments when you didn't trust yourself. Instead of being hard on yourself, check in with yourself. Think about the choices you made and why they may or may not have felt good to you. By being accountable to yourself, you'll gain trust in yourself and in your decision-making ability. You'll also become more confident in being present with your own feelings.

It's okay to feel vulnerable, sad, mad, or embarrassed. Notice your feelings. Breathe. Journal. Do artwork. Talk it out with a friend.

What are you feeling? Where in your body do you feel it? There is no judgment about feelings. They are a part of being human, and your body knows what to do with them. Instead of avoiding feelings or pushing them away, see if you can be with your feelings. Allow them to come over you and then pass. You've got this.

As you recover from stress, you'll be more likely to feel your feelings, and as you feel, you'll become more comfortable with feeling. You'll also be more comfortable being present with a friend or loved one when they have feelings to discuss. And you'll be more willing to take chances and do things you may have never thought you'd do, because you'll know you can handle whatever comes up.

By taking these steps to shift your relationship to yourself and stress, you are shifting your body at a very deep level. You are shifting cortisol and adrenaline production to a level that aligns with healthy function throughout your body. You are making new neural pathways. You are allowing your intestinal lining and leaky gut to heal. You are helping your good gut bacteria to flourish. You are supporting your body so it can digest your food, absorb the nutrients, and use them to make healthy cells. You are helping your mitochondria make energy and hormones. Quite literally, every cell in your body will begin to align with this new way of being.

Like a plant given the right amount of light and darkness, nutrients and hydration, and space and support, you will thrive when given the right components to heal your adrenals from stress and burnout, even though you are still exposed to stress. If and when the stress increases, you'll know to give yourself more support, and support that's specific to your stress type, so you can keep yourself out of stress mode and constantly recovering. Stress recovery is a journey, not a destination. It is something we learn to do as humans, and it allows us to live life as it comes and as we choose.

Please don't feel you are ever doing it "wrong." There is no wrong. There is only being in the moment and noticing how you feel and how your body responds. From there, you can make choices to support your body so it can do what you need it to do.

We all experience stress. That's part of being human. We go through transitions in life. We choose to be parents, to create projects, and to plan events. Miscommunications happen. Relationships come and go. Accidents happen.

And while we attempt to avoid them, betrayals and trauma can happen, too. Our built-in stress response systems and hormones will attempt to protect us. That's when cortisol and adrenaline can go too high or too low, creating the stress types. I think of the stress types as colors in a gradient—one is not better or worse than the other—they are just different variations on a spectrum of possible responses to stress.

How we choose to support ourselves with stress recovery is up to us. Do we feel overwhelmed and victimized by stress and what happens to us? Sometimes this is part of the stress recovery process. Do we then stand back, take a look at the reality we face, and choose to love ourselves, forgive ourselves, and find a way to support ourselves—our bodies, minds, and spirits—so we can recover from the stress exposure?

That's what I refer to as "mastering stress." It involves gaining enough understanding of which stresses can affect us, how our bodies naturally respond, and what we can choose to do on a regular basis to assist recovery. To do this, you have to first find, know, and appreciate yourself inside your body, mind, and spirit and choose to take care of yourself first and foremost.

In this book we've covered each of these aspects of mastering stress so that you can be the master of your stress and your health. No matter where you are starting from, or which stress type you identify with, there is a path to recovery. It involves implementing the C.A.R.E. method on a daily basis, including dietary choices, adequate sleep, stress recovery activities, and exercise that fits you and your stress type. It also involves following the Stress Recovery Protocol phase by phase in order to get out of stress mode, rebalance what got out of balance, and then establish routines in your life to maintain your resilience to stress, for whatever may come along.

Once you've recovered from stress and mastered resiliency, you are in the position to make wise and careful choices about which stresses you keep in your life and how much stress recovery you need. You can become intentional about what you do and experience. And that intentionality will shift the way you interact with your loved ones and community. You will be spreading a sense of mastery of stress, which will help others know it's possible.

Thank you so much for trusting me and joining me on this journey of understanding your body and what you can do to change your health and life, now and in the future. It pleases me and warms my heart to know that I may have been able to help you in even a small way. Blessings to you on your journey.

# Appendix

## Fourteen Recipes to Support Your Body

These easy recipes are appropriate for all stress types. They are dairy-, gluten-, and egg-free, apart from a few recipes in which I suggest butter. (Even though butter is made from cow's milk, it does not tend to trigger food reactions; if you know you can't have butter, I recommend ghee, olive oil, or avocado oil.) For the oil in recipes, I recommend using avocado or grapeseed oil when heating the oil, and extra-virgin olive oil when not heating the oil. When using a dairy-free product (milk or yogurt), choose the type that matches best for your body. Use filtered water, when called for, and sea salt instead of regular salt. I recommend choosing organic ingredients as often as possible. Also choose free-range, hormone-free, antibiotic-free, and non-GMO (non–genetically modified) products.

Be sure to check the ingredient list on the back of any packaged items to be sure they contain no added sugar, high-fructose corn syrup, or artificial sweeteners, which can be listed as cane sugar, sucralose, and dextrose. Avoid artificial colors, preservatives, and natural flavors, which contain chemicals.

# Healing Shake

## • Serves 2 •

This is the pea protein shake I have every morning to keep my blood sugar stable and to get dairy-free, egg-free protein before I work out and start my day. I also like to add in leaky gut healing ingredients and healthy fats. As part of my routine, I take my morning supplements along with my shake. This recipe can easily be customized to suit your taste. Keep it simple or get creative, as you desire.

## Ingredients

- 2 cups water or dairy-free milk (almond, coconut, and/or oat, for example)
- 1 scoop (¼ cup) pea protein powder
- 2 teaspoons collagen powder

- 2 teaspoons leaky gut support powder (ingredients are glutamine, DGL, aloe, arabinogalactan, stevia)
- 2 teaspoons flaxseed oil (or MCT [medium-chain triglyceride] or other desired oil)

## Optional Additions

- ½ cup ice cubes
- ½ cup frozen wild blueberries or raspberries **or** 2 teaspoons liquid berry extract (Proberry)
- ½ avocado, cut in pieces

- ¼ cup nut butter, such as cashew or almond
- ½–1 teaspoon cocoa powder, ground cinnamon, vanilla extract, or ground cardamom

1. Pour the water or milk into the cup of your blender. Add the pea protein, collagen powder, leaky gut healing powder, flaxseed oil, and any desired optional additions.
2. Blend for 30 to 60 seconds. Pour into two drinking glasses and enjoy.

# Gluten-Free Granola or Muesli
### • Serves 4 •

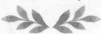

Top this delicious and filling grain-free cereal with fruit and dairy-free milk or yogurt. If you don't know the difference, muesli is served raw and unsweetened, whereas granola is first baked with oil and honey or syrup for a touch of sweetness. You may be surprised at how easy it is to make your own muesli and granola from scratch—in fact, you might want to double the recipe to have cereal on hand for a quick go-to breakfast. If you're in a pinch, you can purchase premade gluten- and grain-free muesli or granola for this recipe. You may also choose to add ½ cup gluten-free rolled oats.

## Ingredients

- ¼ cup almonds
- ¼ cup walnuts
- ¼ cup pecans
- ¼ cup pumpkin seeds
- ¼ cup sunflower seeds
- ¼ cup shredded coconut or carrot
- ½ cup gluten-free rolled oats (optional)

## Additional for Granola

- ½ cup coconut oil
- ½ cup honey or maple syrup
- ½ teaspoon ground cinnamon

## To Serve

- 2 cups dairy-free yogurt or milk (almond, coconut, and/or oat, for example)
- 1 cup frozen wild blueberries, fresh berries, or chopped nectarines
- ¼ cup flaxseed oil (optional)

## For Muesli:

1. Combine the almonds, walnuts, pecans, seeds, coconut or carrot, and rolled oats, if using, in a large bowl. If you're planning to use your muesli later, transfer the mixture to an airtight container and store for up to a month. (If you're serving all the muesli immediately, you can add the dairy-free milk or yogurt to the serving bowl and stir to combine.)
2. To serve, place ½–¾ cup muesli in each bowl and top with ½ cup yogurt or milk, ¼ cup berries or nectarines, and anything else you desire.

## For Granola:

1. Preheat the oven to 425°F. Line a baking sheet with parchment paper.
2. In a large bowl, mix together the almonds, walnuts, pecans, seeds, coconut or carrot, coconut oil, honey or maple syrup, and cinnamon until well combined. Place the mixture on the prepared baking sheet and spread it out evenly.
3. Bake for about 20 minutes, until browning lightly. Remove from the oven and cool for about 10 minutes.
4. Break up the granola into chunks and pieces using a spatula and your hands. If you're planning to use your granola later, let it cool completely, then transfer to an airtight container and store for up to a month.
5. To serve, place ½ to ¾ cup granola in each bowl and top with ½ cup yogurt or milk, ¼ cup berries or nectarines, 1 tablespoon flaxseed oil, if using, and anything else you desire.

# Special Day Pancakes or Waffles
## • Serves 4 •

This gut-friendly gluten-free recipe is perfect for mornings when you have a craving for pancakes or waffles. This recipe offers you two options: you can make it easy by using a premade pancake mix, or you can prepare the batter from scratch using a 1:1 ratio of rice flour and oat flour.

## Ingredients

- 1 cup gluten-free pancake mix **or** ½ cup rice flour plus ½ cup oat flour
- 1 teaspoon baking soda (only if not in premade mix)
- ½ teaspoon sea salt (only if not in premade mix)
- ½ teaspoon ground cinnamon or cardamom (optional)
- ¼ cup avocado or grapeseed oil, plus 1 tablespoon for skillet
- 1 teaspoon vanilla extract
- 2–4 tablespoons water

## To Serve

- ½–1 tablespoon butter for each pancake/waffle
- 1 tablespoon nut butter for each pancake/waffle
- 1 tablespoon maple syrup or honey for each pancake/waffle
- ½ cup fresh fruit or berries
- ¼–½ cup dairy-free cream or yogurt (optional)

1. In a medium bowl, mix the gluten-free pancake mix or flours with the baking soda and sea salt (if not in the premade mix) until thoroughly blended. Add cinnamon or cardamom if desired. Add ¼ cup of the oil and the vanilla. Slowly, while stirring, add just enough water to get the desired consistency. If you prefer thicker pancakes/waffles, add less water. If you prefer crispier pancakes/waffles, add more water until the batter is thin.

2. **For pancakes:** Heat the remaining 1 tablespoon oil in a large skillet over medium heat until it is shiny. Use a spoon to scoop about ¼-cup portions of batter into the pan, making pancakes one by one. It can be fun to make unique shapes like

hearts, flowers, or a mouse head with ears. Cook until the tops of the pancakes are bubbly, then flip and cook them until done—about 2 or 3 minutes on each side. Repeat with the remaining batter.

**For waffles:** Oil and heat a waffle iron according to the manufacturer's directions. Spoon some batter into the waffle iron and close (follow the manufacturer's directions for measuring your batter and cooking the waffle). Open the waffle iron and remove the waffle when it has reached the desired doneness. Repeat with the remaining batter.

3. Serve the pancakes or waffles with butter, nut butter, maple syrup or honey, fresh fruit or berries, and dairy-free cream or yogurt, if desired.

# Colorful Start to the Day

## • Serves 4 •

Breakfast potatoes with onion, peppers, zucchini, mushrooms, greens, and fresh herbs are an amazing way to start the day. Add turkey sausage or bacon for protein. If you have them, you can even use leftovers from the Mexican Ground Turkey (page 238) and/or Your Favorite Roasted Vegetables (page 229) recipes to bring this dish together in a snap.

## Ingredients

- ½ cup chopped spinach or kale
- 1 teaspoon plus 1 pinch of sea salt
- 1–2 tablespoons avocado or grapeseed oil
- ½ medium yellow or red onion, diced
- 1 cup chopped sweet bell peppers (any color)
- 1 medium zucchini, chopped or diced
- ½ cup chopped or sliced mushrooms (shitake, cremini, or baby bella)

- 1 tablespoon chopped fresh rosemary (or 1 teaspoon dried)
- 2 cups chopped and roasted yellow, brown, or red potatoes (or leftover Your Favorite Roasted Vegetables, page 229)
- 1 cup cooked and chopped turkey sausage or bacon (or leftover Mexican Ground Turkey, page 238)

1. Heat a large skillet over medium heat. Add the spinach or kale, a small amount of water, and 1 pinch of the sea salt and sauté until the greens are just wilted. Remove from the pan and set aside.
2. Heat the oil in the same skillet. Add the onion and cook, stirring, until softened, about 2 minutes.
3. Add the bell peppers, zucchini, mushrooms, remaining 1 teaspoon sea salt, and rosemary. Cook, stirring occasionally, until the vegetables are tender and starting to brown, 10–12 minutes.
4. Add the potatoes (or leftover Your Favorite Roasted Vegetables), turkey sausage or bacon (or leftover Mexican Ground Turkey), and wilted greens. Cook for another 2–4 minutes, until slightly browned and warmed through. Transfer to a platter or plate and serve immediately.

# When in Doubt, Arugula!

## • Serves 4 •

Arugula salad with beets, avocado, pumpkin seeds, and olives is my go-to for lunch, for dinner—heck, even for breakfast some days. I like to keep these ingredients (or most of them) on hand so I can whip up a salad in no time, and then head out to my porch to eat it in nature.

## Ingredients

- 4 cups arugula
- 1 cup chopped or thinly sliced cooked beets
- 1 avocado, cut in pieces
- 8 ounces skinless, boneless chicken or turkey breasts, roasted or grilled, cut in pieces
- 12–14 pitted green or Kalamata olives
- ½ cup pumpkin and/or sunflower seeds

## *Balsamic-Dijon Vinaigrette*

- ¼ cup extra-virgin olive oil
- ¼ cup balsamic vinegar
- 1 tablespoon Dijon mustard

1. Divide the arugula among 4 individual serving bowls. Set the beets on the arugula in one area of each bowl. Then set the avocado in another area. Put the chicken or turkey in another area of the bowl. Then evenly space out the olives and sprinkle the seeds over the top of the salad.
2. For the vinaigrette, in a small bowl, whisk together the oil, vinegar, and mustard for 1 minute, until well combined and smooth. Drizzle over each salad.

# Your Favorite Roasted Vegetables

### • Serves 4, or more, depending on how many veggies you include •

You might want to include all of these vegetables or just pick one or two you like and use extra to get to about 3½ pounds total. It's up to you! This dish can be used as an appetizer or side dish, and the leftovers can be used for breakfast or lunch by adding a protein. Choose the seasoning blend you like—I've given you a spicier and a milder option here.

## Ingredients

- 1 large bunch asparagus (about 1 pound) (optional)
- 1 medium head broccoli, cut into florets (optional)
- 1 medium head cauliflower, cut into florets (optional)
- ½ pound brussels sprouts, halved (optional)
- ½ pound multicolor carrots, halved lengthwise then crosswise (optional)
- ½ pound potatoes (yellow, brown, or red), sweet potatoes, or yams, quartered (optional)
- 4 garlic cloves, smashed and peeled, **or** 1 small onion, chopped (optional)
- 2 tablespoons avocado or grapeseed oil

## *Seasoning Blend Options*

### Milder:
- 1 teaspoon garlic powder
- ½ teaspoon dried parsley
- ¼ teaspoon ground black pepper
- ½ teaspoon sea salt

### Spicer:
- 1 teaspoon ground cumin
- ½ teaspoon paprika
- ¼ teaspoon cayenne pepper
- ½ teaspoon sea salt

## *Lemon-Herb Vinaigrette*

- 3 tablespoons fresh lemon juice
- 2 tablespoons extra-virgin olive oil
- ¼ teaspoon sea salt
- ¼ teaspoon ground black pepper

- 2 scallions (white and green parts), sliced
- 3 tablespoons chopped fresh flat-leaf parsley
- ½ cup dairy-free cheese (optional)

1. Preheat the oven to 425° F.
2. Place the vegetables (including the garlic or onion if desired) on a 13 × 9-inch baking pan or rimmed sheet pan. Drizzle with the oil and toss to coat.
3. To make the seasoning blend, combine the spices and sea salt in a small bowl. Sprinkle the seasoning blend over the vegetables and toss again, then spread into an even layer in the pan.
4. Roast, giving the pan a shake or stir about halfway through, for 35–40 minutes, until the veggies are tender (if you're using potatoes, the cooking time may be longer).
5. Toward the end of the cooking time, make the vinaigrette. In a small bowl, whisk together the lemon juice, oil, sea salt, and pepper. Stir in the scallions, parsley, and dairy-free cheese, if desired.
6. Arrange the vegetables on a serving plate and spoon the vinaigrette over the top.

# Simply Quinoa

· **Makes 3 cups cooked quinoa (serves 4 people ¾ cup)** ·

A common substitute for rice, quinoa is actually a seed that is higher in protein than most grains. You can eat this quinoa as a side to a meal or add to it to greens for a quinoa salad.

## Ingredients

· 1 cup quinoa

· 2 cups filtered water

1. In a medium saucepan, combine the quinoa with the water and bring to a boil over medium-high heat. Stir once, cover with a tight-fitting lid, and reduce the heat to medium-low. Cook for 12–15 minutes, until the water is absorbed.
2. Remove from the heat and fluff with a fork. Let stand covered for 5 minutes more, then serve in a bowl or use in another recipe.

# Bowls of Goodness
## • Serves 4 •

Loaded with protein and fresh veggies, these bowls are endlessly customizable and an easy, satisfying lunch or dinner. Choose chicken, turkey, or chickpeas. Layer over quinoa with spinach, avocado, grapes, and lemon vinaigrette. Or go for rice noodles, cabbage, red pepper, scallions, and lime vinaigrette . . . depending on your mood. You can't go wrong!

## Ingredients

- 2 cups spinach leaves **or** ½ medium head green cabbage, shredded
- 2 cups cooked quinoa **or** 2 cups thin rice noodles, cooked and cooled
- 1 (6- to 8-ounce) skinless, boneless chicken or turkey breast, cooked, **or** 1 (15-ounce) can chickpeas, rinsed and drained
- ½ cucumber, sliced into half-moons
- 1 avocado, diced, **or** 4 scallions (white and green parts), sliced
- 1 cup chopped grapes, slivered almonds, or pomegranate seeds, **or** 1 cup thinly sliced red bell pepper

## Simplest Citrus Vinaigrette

- ¼ cup extra-virgin olive oil
- ¼ cup fresh lemon or lime juice (from about 2 lemons or limes)
- ½ teaspoon sea salt

## To Serve

- Chopped fresh parsley or basil (optional, for a garnish)

1. Divide the spinach or cabbage and quinoa or rice noodles among 4 bowls. Add the chicken, turkey, or chickpeas; cucumber; avocado or scallions; and grapes,

almonds, pomegranate seeds, or red pepper. Or you can layer the ingredients of your choice in a large serving bowl.

2. For the vinaigrette, in a small bowl, whisk together the oil, lemon or lime juice, and sea salt. Drizzle over each salad. If desired, sprinkle parsley or basil on each salad.

# Roasted Chicken or Turkey with Herbs (Plus Broth)
## • Serves 4 •

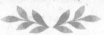

While this recipe can be used for a holiday meal, I find that it can be a great recipe to use anytime, especially if you are cooking for a family. The poultry can be served for dinner and used again for lunch, on a salad or in a sandwich. Reserve the bones to use as the start of a soup or bone broth—see the note that follows the recipe.

## Ingredients

- 2 carrots
- 2 celery stalks
- 1 large onion
- 6 tablespoons butter, softened, or avocado or grapeseed oil, divided
- 1 whole chicken or turkey (about 5 pounds)
- 1 lemon, quartered

- 2 tablespoons chopped fresh thyme leaves (or ½ teaspoon dried)
- 2 tablespoons chopped fresh sage (or ½ teaspoon dried)
- 1 tablespoon chopped fresh rosemary (or ¼ teaspoon dried)
- 1 teaspoon sea salt
- ¼ teaspoon ground black pepper
- 2 tablespoons rice flour

1. Preheat the oven to 425°F.
2. Finely dice the carrots, celery, and onion (to make a mirepoix).
3. In a skillet or in the roasting pan you plan to use, melt 2 tablespoons of the butter or heat the oil over medium-low heat. Add the diced vegetables and cook, stirring occasionally, for about 10 minutes, until the onion is translucent. Your goal is just to soften the vegetables, so decrease the heat if needed to avoid browning. If you cooked the veggies in a skillet, transfer them to the bottom of the roasting pan.
4. Place the chicken or turkey in the roasting pan. Place the lemon inside the cavity or in the pan.
5. Place the remaining 4 tablespoons butter or oil in a small bowl and mix in the herbs, sea salt, and pepper. Spread the butter mixture over the surface of the chicken or turkey. Put any extra in the bottom of the pan.

6. Roast the chicken or turkey for 15 minutes. Then reduce the temperature to 350°F and roast, basting every 8–12 minutes, for an additional 2–2½ hours, or until a meat thermometer placed in the thickest area reads 165°F. When cutting, there should be no traces of pink. Transfer the chicken or turkey to a plate, cover, and let rest for 10 minutes.

7. Place the roasting pan (with the mirepoix and juices) over low heat. Add the rice flour while whisking and simmer until the mixture thickens into a roux. If there are not enough juices, add ½–¾ cup water. Taste to see if the gravy needs more sea salt and pepper, and season as needed. Strain the gravy, if desired, or leave the mirepoix in and blend with a hand mixer or immersion blender until it is smooth. Pour into a gravy boat or bowl for serving.

8. To carve the chicken or turkey, place on a clean cutting board. Using a knife and fork, cut between the breast and the wing. Remove the wing and cut the breast into slices. Then cut the legs from the body to make leg and thigh portions. Serve with the gravy or cut into chunks to use in another recipe.

Note: Once the meat is carved, the bones can be used to make a broth. Place the bones in a large pot and cover with water. You may add 1 or 2 tablespoons apple cider vinegar or lemon juice, and flavor your broth with onion, garlic, celery, carrots, rosemary, and/or parsley. Bring to a boil, then reduce the heat and simmer for at least 2 hours (for soup broth) or 10–12 hours (for bone broth). Strain and use immediately or freeze for later.

# Pan-Roasted Herb Chicken or Turkey Breasts with Savory Sauce

## • Serves 4 •

Having a go-to recipe for chicken or turkey breasts makes all the difference in your self-care routine. You can pair this chicken or turkey with vegetables or a salad, save it for lunch tomorrow, or use it in a soup.

## Ingredients

- 4 (6- to 8-ounce) skinless, boneless chicken or turkey breasts, whole or cut into tenders
- ½ teaspoon sea salt
- 2 tablespoons fresh rosemary or sage leaves (or 1 teaspoon dried)
- 1 tablespoon fresh thyme leaves (or 1½ teaspoons dried)

- 2–3 tablespoons avocado or grapeseed oil
- 4 garlic cloves, smashed, peeled, and chopped
- ½ cup fresh orange juice, apple cider, or balsamic vinegar
- ½ cup chicken broth (or 2 tablespoons water and 4 tablespoons cold butter)

1. Pat the chicken or turkey breasts dry with paper towels. Sprinkle the sea salt on both sides. In a small bowl, combine the herbs.

2. Heat 2 tablespoons of the oil in a large skillet over medium-high heat. Put the chicken in the hot skillet and sprinkle with half of the herbs. Cook covered and undisturbed, until the undersides are golden brown, about 6 minutes. Turn the chicken over and cook about 6 minutes more, until browned and cooked through (you can cut into the thickest part to make sure it is no longer pink). Transfer to a plate or platter.

3. If the oil in the skillet is used up, add 1 tablespoon more. Add the garlic and cook, stirring, for 1–2 minutes, until golden brown. Stir in the remaining herbs and cook for 30 seconds, until fragrant. Add the orange juice or vinegar to the skillet and bring to a boil, then cook, stirring and scraping up the browned bits, until reduced to about 2 tablespoons, about 4 minutes. Add the chicken broth (or water and butter), reduce heat to low, and simmer for 3–4 minutes more, until the sauce starts to thicken slightly. Taste for salt and add more if necessary. Spoon the sauce over the chicken.

# Meat Sauce with Onions and Herbs

## • Serves 4 •

My daughter loves this recipe over gluten-free pasta, but it can also be served with zucchini noodles, roasted vegetables, or gluten-free bread, or inside rice wraps like spring rolls.

## Ingredients

- 2 tablespoons avocado or grapeseed oil
- ½ medium onion, diced
- 1 or 2 garlic cloves, smashed, peeled, and diced
- 2 pounds ground beef or turkey
- 1 tablespoon chopped fresh oregano (or ½ teaspoon dried)
- 1 tablespoon chopped fresh basil (or ½ teaspoon dried)
- 1½ teaspoons chopped fresh rosemary (or ¼ teaspoon dried)
- 1½ teaspoons chopped fresh thyme (or ¼ teaspoon dried)
- ½ teaspoon sea salt
- 1 (24-ounce) jar marinara sauce

1. Heat the oil in a large skillet over medium heat. Add the onion and garlic, and cook, stirring, until the onion is softened, about 2 minutes. Add the ground beef, herbs, and sea salt. Cook, breaking the beef into small pieces with a spatula, and stir just until brown, 5–6 minutes. Add the marinara while continuing to stir. Cook for 4–5 minutes more, until the sauce is simmering and the beef is fully cooked. Transfer to a serving bowl or use in another recipe.

# Mexican Ground Turkey

## • Serves 4 •

This tasty and flexible ground turkey is perfect in a tostada appetizer, tacos, spring rolls with rice wraps, or my Colorful Start to the Day (page 227). Making your own Mexican/taco seasoning from scratch helps you avoid preservatives and other unwanted ingredients (I was so excited to figure this out!), but if you're in a pinch, feel free to substitute a premade taco seasoning mix (you'll need about 3 tablespoons).

## Ingredients

### Make Your Own Seasoning Blend

- 1 tablespoon ancho chili powder
- 1½ teaspoons ground cumin
- 1 teaspoon sea salt
- ½ teaspoon ground black pepper
- ½ teaspoon paprika
- ¼ teaspoon garlic powder
- ¼ teaspoon onion powder
- ¼ teaspoon red pepper flakes
- ¼ teaspoon dried oregano

### *Mexican Ground Turkey*

- 1 tablespoon avocado or grapeseed oil
- ½ medium yellow onion, chopped
- 1 pound ground turkey
- 1 cup shredded dairy-free cheddar (optional)
- ½ cup chopped fresh cilantro (optional)

1. Mix the seasoning blend ingredients in a small bowl (or have ready about 3 tablespoons of premade taco seasoning mix).
2. For the turkey, heat the oil in a large skillet over medium heat. Add the onion and cook, stirring, until softened, about 2 minutes. Add the ground turkey and cook, breaking it into small pieces with a spatula, and stir until just starting to brown, 3–4 minutes. Sprinkle the seasoning blend over the meat while continuing to stir. Cook for 6–8 minutes more, until fully browned.
3. Transfer to a platter or use in another recipe. Sprinkle the dairy-free cheddar and cilantro, if desired, on top of the meat.

# Grandma's Fruit Pie or Cobbler

## • Serves 4 •

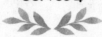

I use essentially this same gluten-free dough to make all kinds of desserts: pies, tarts, cobblers, crumbles, biscuits, and even shortcakes. Often I use apples or berries, but in the summer I love to use peaches or rhubarb. The foundation of this recipe came from both of my grandmothers, whom I consider to be pie experts! I wish I could have them test out my gluten-free recipe with alternative sweeteners—I think they'd love them as much as I do.

## Ingredients

### Gluten-Free Pastry Dough

- 1½ cups gluten-free all-purpose flour *or* ¾ cup rice flour plus ¾ cup oat flour
- ½ teaspoon sea salt
- ½ cup cold salted butter, cut into small pieces
- ⅔ cup water

### Additions for Cobbler

- 1 tablespoon baking powder
- ¼ cup coconut palm sugar, monk fruit, or stevia
- ½ teaspoon ground cinnamon
- ¼ teaspoon ground ginger, cardamom, or allspice (optional)
- ½ teaspoon vanilla extract

## Filling

- 4–6 cups chopped fruit (choose one of the following):
- 8 Granny Smith apples, nectarines, or peaches (or a combination), cut into ½-inch pieces
- 4 cups blueberries, raspberries, or blackberries (or a combination)
- 5–6 rhubarb stalks, cut into ½-inch pieces (optional)
- ½ cup coconut palm sugar, monk fruit, or maple syrup (increase to 1 cup if using rhubarb)
- 2 tablespoons gluten-free all-purpose flour
- 2 tablespoons fresh lemon juice (or can be from a container)
- ½ teaspoon ground cinnamon
- 1 tablespoon butter, cut into pieces

## To Serve

- Dairy-Free Ice Cream (page 241)

1. Preheat the oven to 375°F. If you're making cobbler, lightly butter a baking dish (a pie pan doesn't require buttering).

2. To make the dough, stir together the flour and sea salt (and the baking powder, cinnamon, and spices [if desired] if making cobbler) in a large bowl until mixed evenly. Add the butter and press into the flour mixture using a fork or pastry cutter until the mixture resembles coarse meal. Slowly add just enough water (and the vanilla if making cobbler), stirring just until the dough comes together.

3. If making a pie, use a rolling pin to roll out the dough on a clean, floured surface. You should end up with a round crust that's about an inch wider than your pie pan. Transfer the dough to the pan and use your fingers to flute around the edge. Or you can do what I often do to save time and just press the dough right into the pie pan, without rolling it out. Save some dough to cover the fruit if you'd like.

4. To make the filling, toss together the filling ingredients in a large bowl. For a pie, transfer the filling to the pie pan (on top of the dough in the bottom of the pan), and use extra dough to cover the filling, if desired. For a cobbler, transfer the filling to the buttered baking dish, and place pieces of dough over the top of the filling with the extra dough.

5. Bake at 375°F for about 45 minutes, until the filling is bubbling and the crust is browning. If at any point during baking the crust is browning too much, cover with foil.

6. Carefully remove from the oven and allow to cool for at least 10 minutes. Serve with Dairy-Free Ice Cream (page 241).

# Dairy-Free Ice Cream

## • Serves 4 •

Homemade makes all the difference. This coconut-based ice cream is delicious by itself or with fruit, chopped nuts, or fruit pie. One of my favorite ways to eat it is with frozen wild blueberries, but you can also add the berries right into the ice cream—or make it any other flavor you'd like. I always try to have some protein, even with dessert, so you can use pea protein powder, nuts, or nut butter to add protein.

## Ingredients

- 2 cans full-fat coconut milk
- ½ cup honey
- 1 teaspoon vanilla extract
- ⅛ teaspoon sea salt

## Optional Additions

- 2 tablespoons pea protein powder
- 1–2 tablespoons cocoa powder
- 1 teaspoon ground cinnamon
- ¼ cup fresh or frozen wild blueberries (or other berries)
- 2–3 tablespoons nuts or nut butter

1. Put the cans of coconut milk in the refrigerator and the tub of the ice cream maker in the freezer for 24 hours.
2. In a large bowl, combine the cold coconut milk, honey, and vanilla and stir to mix well. Add the sea salt and any other desired ingredients *except* berries, nuts, and/or nut butter (wait until the ice cream is almost solid to add them).
3. Pour the coconut milk mixture into the tub of the ice cream maker and follow the instruction manual to make the ice cream. Just before it is solid, add berries, nuts, and/or nut butter, if desired.
4. Scoop the ice cream out of the tub and into a freezer container. Serve immediately or put in the freezer to eat later.

# Acknowledgments

Nineteen years ago today (the day I finished this book), I gave birth to my daughter, Ella, at home in New York. It was a culmination of everything I had experienced in my life to that point, including pain and joy. I had learned from doctors, midwives, teachers, women, and my own body, to trust the process, even when it seemed like it was stuck, and to relax more than I thought was possible. To be completely committed to the outcome and yet unattached to how the process looks or happens.

Now today, I realize I am giving birth to this book, after another process of trust, expression, and allowing the process to happen. In these pages, I shared what I have learned through my experiences as a human, a mother, a naturopathic doctor, and midwife, and from my many teachers along the way, including my daughter and my parents.

My father is a pharmacist. Throughout his career he ran a pharmacy, which grew into him managing a whole chain of 1,200 pharmacies. Thinking about it now, I'm impressed by his ability to see the big picture while also connecting and communicating with each person involved in serving the pharmacy's customers. He worked extremely hard (and still does!), is a leader, and sees each project to completion. My mother is a teacher and musician—a flutist, to be specific. Ultimately, I think of her as an artist who makes everything beautiful. She taught me that understanding what we are going through makes it easier. After recovering from a stroke this past year, she spent hours with me in her kitchen as I developed the recipes in this book. So, if anyone ever wondered what you get when you combine a pharmacist and a teacher/artist, the answer is that you get a naturopathic doctor—using food, nutrients, herbs, and mindfulness to help people navigate life. I am eternally grateful to my parents for showing me that even when stress is high and things are changing and difficult, it is possible to find our way through it, to survive and even to thrive.

I am so grateful to everyone who played a role in helping me to create this book to share with others in the hopes that it may help them too. That includes JJ Virgin, with whom I first shared the idea of the stress types, and who encouraged me to write about it. My book agents—Jaidree Braddix and Celeste Fine. Kristina Grish, who helped me with the book proposal. The entire team at BenBella Books, including Glenn Yeffeth and Claire Schulz, my editor. Thank you to Gregory Newton Brown and to Jennifer Brett Greenstein, who helped shape the book and prepare it for all of you. I am also so grateful to Michelle Farinella, my creative director, who helped design the back cover and made sure my voice and message comes through in all marketing of the book.

I would like to give special thanks to Don Gino, my shaman, and Shelley Ruitta, who guided my spiritual growth during the time of writing this book. I would also like to thank Dr. Warren Wilner, a brilliant psychoanalyst who helped me to know myself and for many conversations about the strain caused by stress that causes distress and how we humans can recover.

When writing this book, I had just emerged from an extremely stressful time in my life, when I realized people whom I had trusted to help me were taking advantage of my trust. I also realized I needed to learn how to communicate and choose with more intention. To do that, I needed to know myself better and be clear about what I wanted to create. It was in ceremony with other brave souls, who also wanted to know themselves better and were willing to face whatever was needed in order to find themselves and their purpose in life. I am most grateful to be inspired by all of you. The various physical and emotional stresses I experienced caused a growth on my neck, related to my clavicle (doctors don't have a name for it). After much imaging and several biopsies, we discovered that it was not cancerous, and yet it continued to grow and protrude from my neck. I was reluctant to go through surgery to have it removed, but ultimately realized that was necessary and searched to find a surgeon who was willing to perform the surgery. I'm writing now on the other side of that process, which spanned over two years and coincided with writing this book. I want to acknowledge it here, because I feel grateful to my body for showing me that it was stressed and needed support to recover. My body essentially taught me what I needed to know in order to share the messages in this book.

I feel so much appreciation for my amazing support staff, including Melissa Bellard, Jackie Packman, and Lou Capezza. There are many others who believed in my vision and helped to get it out to readers on social media, DoctorDoni.com, and my podcast, How Humans Heal, including Dr. Heather Paulson, Summer Bock, Theresa Depasquale, Bonnie Mott, Randi Best-Kaye, Michael Boezi, Michelle Bell, Rachael Henning, and Josh Williams. Thank you all for being on this journey with me. Thank you to Dr. Steve Nenninger for many conversations about this book and your encouragement to share my thoughts with readers.

And to my patients, I couldn't have written this book or developed the Stress Recovery Protocol without you. Thank you for trusting me to support you with your health and for sharing your experiences with me so that I could learn from you what could potentially help others too.

# Notes

## Chapter 1

1. Monalisha Sahu and Josyula G. Prasuna, "Twin Studies: A Unique Epidemiological Tool," *Indian Journal of Community Medicine* 41, no. 3 (2016): 177–82, doi:10.4103/0970-0218.183593.
2. Irene Lacal and Rossella Ventura, "Epigenetic Inheritance: Concepts, Mechanisms, and Perspectives," *Frontiers in Molecular Neuroscience* (September 28, 2018): 11, doi:10.3389/fnmol.2018.00292.
3. Leonard W. Poon et al., "Understanding Centenarians' Psychosocial Dynamics and Their Contributions to Health and Quality of Life," *Current Gerontology and Geriatrics Research* 2010 (September 26, 2010): 680657, doi:10.1155/2010/680657; Marirosa Dello Buono, Ornella Urciuoli, and Diego de Leo, "Quality of Life and Longevity: A Study of Centenarians," *Age and Ageing* 27, no. 2 (March 1998): 207–16, doi:10.1093/ageing/27.2.207; Donald Craig Willcox, Bradley J. Willcox, and Leonard W. Poon, "Centenarian Studies: Important Contributors to Our Understanding of the Aging Process and Longevity," *Current Gerontology and Geriatrics Research* 2010 (July 13, 2011): 484529, doi:10.1155/2010/484529.
4. Abiola Keller et al., "Does the Perception That Stress Affects Health Matter? The Association with Health and Mortality," *Health Psychology* 31, no. 5 (2012): 677–84, doi:10.1037/a0026743.
5. Neil Schneiderman, Gail Ironson, and Scott D. Siegel, "Stress and Health: Psychological, Behavioral, and Biological Determinants," *Annual Review of Clinical Psychology* 1 (April 27, 2005): 607–28, doi:10.1146/annurev.clinpsy.1.102803.144141.
6. Sean M. Smith and Wylie W. Vale, "The Role of the Hypothalamic-Pituitary-Adrenal Axis in Neuroendocrine Responses to Stress," *Dialogues in Clinical Neuroscience* 8, no. 4 (2006): 383–95, doi:10.31887/DCNS.2006.8.4/ssmith.
7. Donielle Wilson, "Anxiety and Depression: It All Starts with Stress," *Integrative Medicine* 8, no. 3 (June/July 2009): 42–5.
8. Marilia Carabotti et al., "The Gut-Brain Axis: Interactions Between Enteric Microbiota, Central and Enteric Nervous Systems," *Annals of Gastroenterology* 28, no. 2 (April–June 2015): 203–9, https://pubmed.ncbi.nlm.nih.gov/25830558/.

9. John R. Kelly et al., "Breaking Down the Barriers: The Gut Microbiome, Intestinal Permeability and Stress-Related Psychiatric Disorders," *Frontiers in Cellular Neuroscience* (October 14, 2015), doi:10.3389/fncel.2015.00392.
10. Micaela Rodriguez, Benjamin W. Bellet, and Richard J. McNally, "Reframing Time Spent Alone: Reappraisal Buffers the Emotional Effects of Isolation," *Cognitive Therapy and Research* 44 (2020):1–16, doi:10.1007/s10608-020-10128-x.
11. Mark P. Mattson, "Hormesis Defined," *Ageing Research Reviews* 7, no. 1 (January 2008): 1–7, doi:10.1016/j.arr.2007.08.007.
12. Peramaiyan Rajendran et al., "Autophagy and Senescence: A New Insight in Selected Human Diseases," *Journal of Cellular Physiology* (May 29, 2019), doi:10.1002/jcp.28895.
13. Éric Le Bourg, "Hormesis, Aging, and Longevity," *Biochimica et Biophysica Acta (BBA)—General Subjects* 1790, no. 10 (October 2009): 1030–9, doi:10.1016/j.bbagen.2009.01.004.
14. Keller et al., "Does the Perception That Stress Affects Health Matter?"

## Chapter 2

1. Dr. Doni Wilson, *The Stress Remedy: Master Your Body's Synergy and Optimize Your Health* (Empowering Wellness Press, 2013).
2. Judith A. Lothian, "Do Not Disturb: The Importance of Privacy in Labor," *Journal of Perinatal Education* 13, no. 3 (2004): 4–6, doi:10.1624/105812404X1707.
3. Hans Selye, "Forty Years of Stress Research: Principal Remaining Problems and Misconceptions," *Canadian Medical Association Journal* 115, no. 1 (July 3, 1976): 53–6, https://www.ncbi.nlm.nih.gov/pmc/articles/PMC1878603/.
4. Lotte Gerritsen et al., "HPA Axis Genes, and Their Interaction with Childhood Maltreatment, Are Related to Cortisol Levels and Stress-Related Phenotypes," *Neuropsychopharmacology* 42 (June 7, 2017): 2446–55, doi:10.1038/npp.2017.118.
5. Ho Jang Kwon, Han Jun Jin, and Myung Ho Lim, "Association Between *Monoamine Oxidase* Gene Polymorphisms and Attention Deficit Hyperactivity Disorder in Korean Children," *Genetic Testing and Molecular Biomarkers* 18, no. 7 (July 11, 2014), doi:10.1089/gtmb.2014.0066; Mohammad Reza Eslami Amirabadi et al., "Monoamine Oxidase A Gene Polymorphisms and Bipolar Disorder in Iranian Population," *Iranian Red Crescent Medical Journal* 17, no. 2 (February 2015): e23095, https://www.ncbi.nlm.nih.gov/pmc/articles/PMC4353216/; Różycka Agata et al., "The *MAOA, COMT, MTHFR* and *ESR1* Gene Polymorphisms Are Associated with the Risk of Depression in Menopausal Women," *Maturitas* 84 (February 1, 2016): 42–54, doi:10.1016/j.maturitas.2015.10.011.
6. Charles E. Griffin, III et al., "Benzodiazepine Pharmacology and Central Nervous System–Mediated Effects," *Ochsner Journal* 13, no. 2 (Summer 2013): 214–23, https://www.ncbi.nlm.nih.gov/pmc/articles/PMC3684331/.

## Chapter 3

1. Tarani Chandola et al., "Are Flexible Work Arrangements Associated with Lower Levels of Chronic Stress-Related Biomarkers? A Study of 6025 Employees in the UK Household Longitudinal Study," *Sociology* 53, no. 4 (2019): 779–99, doi:10.1177/0038038519826014.

2. Vincent J Felitti et al., "Relationship of Childhood Abuse and Household Dysfunction to Many of the Leading Causes of Death in Adults: The Adverse Childhood Experiences (ACE) Study," *American Journal of Preventive Medicine* 14, no. 4 (May 1, 1998): 245–58, doi:10.1016/S0749-3797(98)00017-8.

3. William E. Copeland et al., "Traumatic Events and Posttraumatic Stress in Childhood," *Archives of General Psychiatry* 64, no. 5 (May 2007): 577–84, doi:10.1001/arch psyc.64.5.577.

4. Christina Bethell et al., "Positive Childhood Experiences and Adult Mental and Relational Health in a Statewide Sample: Associations Across Adverse Childhood Experiences Levels," *JAMA Pediatrics* 173, no. 11 (2019): e193007, doi:10.1001/jama pediatrics.2019.3007.

5. Oscar F. Garcia et al., "Parenting Warmth and Strictness Across Three Generations: Parenting Styles and Psychosocial Adjustment," *International Journal of Environmental Research and Public Health* 17, no. 20 (October 15, 2020): 7487, doi:10.3390 /ijerph17207487; Keith A. King, Rebecca A. Vidourek, and Ashley L. Merianos, "Authoritarian Parenting and Youth Depression: Results from a National Study," *Journal of Prevention & Intervention in the Community* 44, no. 2 (2016): 130–9, doi :10.1080/10852352.2016.1132870; Esther Calzada et al., "Early Childhood Internalizing Problems in Mexican- and Dominican-Origin Children: The Role of Cultural Socialization and Parenting Practices," *Journal of Clinical Child & Adolescent Psychology* 46, no. 4 (2017): 551–62, doi:10.1080/15374416.2015.1041593.

6. Maria A. Gartstein and Michael K. Skinner, "Prenatal Influences on Temperament Development: The Role of Environmental Epigenetics," *Development and Psychopathology* 30, no. 4 (2018): 1269–303, doi:10.1017/S0954579417001730; Mallory E. Bowers and Rachel Yehuda, "Intergenerational Transmission of Stress in Humans," *Neuropsychopharmacology* 41 (2016): 232–44, doi:10.1038/npp.2015.247.

7. Maria A. Gartstein and Michael K. Skinner, "Prenatal Influences on Temperament Development: The Role of Environmental Epigenetics," *Developmental Psychopathology* 30, no. 4 (2018): 1269–303, doi:10.1017/S0954579417001730; Shizhao Li et al., "Prenatal Epigenetics Diets Play Protective Roles Against Environmental Pollution," *Clinical Epigenetics* 11 (May 16, 2019): 82, doi:10.1186/s13148-019-0659-4.

8. Hari Sharma, "Meditation: Process and Effects," *AYU* 36 (2015): 233–7, doi:10 .4103/0974-8520.182756.

9. Haitao Guo, Justin B Callaway, and Jenny P-Y Ting, "Inflammasomes: Mechanism of Action, Role in Disease, and Therapeutics," *Nature Medicine* 21 (June 29, 2015): 677–87, doi:10.1038/nm.3893.

10. Michael Ristow and Kathrin Schmeisser, "Mitohormesis: Promoting Health and Lifespan by Increased Levels of Reactive Oxygen Species (ROS)," *Dose-Response* 12, no. 2 (April 1, 2014): doi:10.2203/dose-response.13-035.Ristow.

11. Wendy R. Hood et al., "Life History Trade-Offs within the Context of Mitochondrial Hormesis," *Integrative and Comparative Biology* 58, no. 3 (September 2018): 567–77, doi:10.1093/icb/icy073.

12. Chen Chen et al., "The Microbiota Continuum Along the Female Reproductive Tract and Its Relation to Uterine-Related Diseases," *Nature Communications* 8 (October 17, 2017): 875, doi:10.1038/s41467-017-00901-0.

13. Joe Alcock, Carlo C. Maley, and C. Athena Aktipis, "Is Eating Behavior Manipulated by the Gastrointestinal Microbiota? Evolutionary Pressures and Potential Mechanisms," *BioEssays* 36, no. 10 (October 2014): 940–9, doi:10.1002/bies.201400071.

14. Michael A. Conlon and Anthony R. Bird, "The Impact of Diet and Lifestyle on Gut Microbiota and Human Health," *Nutrients* 7, no. 1 (December 24, 2014): 17–44, doi:10.3390/nu7010017.

15. Luc Biedermann and Gerhard Rogler, "The Intestinal Microbiota: Its Role in Health and Disease," *European Journal of Pediatrics* 174 (January 7, 2015): 151–67, doi:10.1007/s00431-014-2476-2; Rui Liu et al., "Dysbiosis of Gut Microbiota Associated with Clinical Parameters in Polycystic Ovary Syndrome," *Frontiers in Microbiology* 8 (February 28, 2017): 324, doi:10.3389/fmicb.2017.00324; Ana López-Moreno and Margarita Aguilera, "Probiotics Dietary Supplementation for Modulating Endocrine and Fertility Microbiota Dysbiosis," *Nutrients* 12, no. 3 (March 13, 2020): 757, doi:10.3390/nu12030757; Carra A. Simpson et al., "Feeling Down? A Systematic Review of the Gut Microbiota in Anxiety/Depression and Irritable Bowel Syndrome," *Journal of Affective Disorders* 266 (April 1, 2020): 429–46, doi:10.1016/j.jad.2020.01.124; G. Adrienne Weiss and Thierry Hennet, "Mechanisms and Consequences of Intestinal Dysbiosis," *Cellular and Molecular Life Sciences* 74 (2017): 2959–77, doi:10.1007/s00018-017-2509-x.

16. J. Philip Karl et al., "Effects of Psychological, Environmental and Physical Stressors on the Gut Microbiota," *Frontiers in Microbiology* 9 (September 11, 2018): 2013, doi:10.3389/fmicb.2018.02013; Philip Strandwitz, "Neurotransmitter Modulation by the Gut Microbiota," *Brain Research* 1693B (August 15, 2018): 128–33, doi:10.1016/j.brainres.2018.03.015.

17. Ricard Farré et al., "Intestinal Permeability, Inflammation and the Role of Nutrients," *Nutrients* 12, no. 4 (April 23, 2020): 1185, doi:10.3390/nu12041185.

18. Marilia Carabotti et al., "The Gut-Brain Axis: Interactions Between Enteric Microbiota, Central and Enteric Nervous Systems," *Annals of Gastroenterology* 28, no. 2 (April–June 2015): 203–9, https://pubmed.ncbi.nlm.nih.gov/25830558/.

19. Laurie H. Glimcher and Ann-Hwee Lee, "From Sugar to Fat: How the Transcription Factor XBP1 Regulates Hepatic Lipogenesis," *Annals of the New York Academy of Sciences* 1173, no. s1 (September 2009): E2–9, doi:10.1111/j.1749-6632.2009.04956.x.

20. Michael Irwin et al., "Effects of Sleep and Sleep Deprivation on Catecholamine and Interleukin-2 Levels in Humans: Clinical Implications," *Journal of Clinical Endocrinology & Metabolism* 84, no. 6 (June 1, 1999): 1979–85, doi:10.1210/jcem.84.6.5788.

## Chapter 4

1. S. Nenninger, phone conversation about Wu Wei, December 8, 2020.

2. Athanasios Valavanidis, Thomais Vlachogianni, and Constantinos Fiotakis, "8-hydroxy-2' -deoxyguanosine (8-OHdG): A Critical Biomarker of Oxidative Stress and Carcinogenesis," *Journal of Environmental Science and Health, Part C* 27, no. 2 (May 1, 2009): 120–39, doi:10.1080/10590500902885684.

## Chapter 6

1. Ann F. La Berge, "How the Ideology of Low Fat Conquered America," *Journal of the History of Medicine and Allied Sciences* 63, no. 2 (April 2008): 139–77, doi:10.1093/jhmas/jrn001.

2.  Barbara V. Howard et al., "Low-Fat Dietary Pattern and Risk of Cardiovascular Disease: The Women's Health Initiative Randomized Controlled Dietary Modification Trial," *JAMA* 295, no. 6 (2006): 655–66, doi:10.1001/jama.295.6.655.

3.  American Diabetes Association, "Lifestyle Management: Standards of Medical Care in Diabetes—2019," *Diabetes Care* 42 supplement 1 (January 2019): S46–60, doi:10.2337/dc19-S005.

4.  Luc Tappy, "Basics in Clinical Nutrition: Carbohydrate Metabolism," *Clinical Nutrition Aspen* 3, no. 5 (October 1, 2008): E192–5, doi:10.1016/j.eclnm.2008.06.010.

5.  Celia Martinez-Perez et al., "Use of Different Food Classification Systems to Assess the Association Between Ultra-Processed Food Consumption and Cardiometabolic Health in an Elderly Population with Metabolic Syndrome (PREDIMED-Plus Cohort)," *Nutrients* 13, no. 7 (July 20, 2021): 2471, doi:10.3390/nu13072471.

6.  Justin Hollon et al., "Effect of Gliadin on Permeability of Intestinal Biopsy Explants from Celiac Disease Patients and Patients with Non-Celiac Gluten Sensitivity," *Nutrients* 7, no. 3 (February 27, 2015): 1565–76, doi:10.3390/nu7031565; Victor F. Zevallos et al., "Nutritional Wheat Amylase-Trypsin Inhibitors Promote Intestinal Inflammation via Activation of Myeloid Cells," *Gastroenterology* 152, no. 5 (April 1, 2017): 1100–13, doi:10.1053/j.gastro.2016.12.006.

7.  Conor P Kerley, "A Review of Plant-Based Diets to Prevent and Treat Heart Failure," *Cardiac Failure Review* 4, no. 1 (2018): 54–61, doi:10.15420/cfr.2018:1:1; Hyunju Kim et al., "Plant-Based Diets Are Associated with a Lower Risk of Incident Cardiovascular Disease, Cardiovascular Disease Mortality, and All-Cause Mortality in a General Population of Middle-Aged Adults," *Journal of the American Heart Association* 8, no. 16 (2019): e012865, doi:10.1161/JAHA.119.012865.

8.  Winston J. Craig, "Health Effects of Vegan Diets," *American Journal of Clinical Nutrition* 89, no. 5 (May 2009): 1627S–33S, doi:10.3945/ajcn.2009.26736N; Hercules Sakkas et al., "Nutritional Status and the Influence of the Vegan Diet on the Gut Microbiota and Human Health," *Medicina* 56, no. 2 (February 19, 2020): 88, doi:10.3390/medicina56020088.

9.  Stijn Soenen et al., "Normal Protein Intake Is Required for Body Weight Loss and Weight Maintenance, and Elevated Protein Intake for Additional Preservation of Resting Energy Expenditure and Fat Free Mass," *Journal of Nutrition* 143, no. 5 (May 2013): 591–6, doi:10.3945/jn.112.167593.

10. Marta Lonnie et al., "Protein for Life: Review of Optimal Protein Intake, Sustainable Dietary Sources and the Effect on Appetite in Ageing Adults," *Nutrients* 10, no. 3 (March 14, 2018): 360, doi:10.3390/nu10030360.

11. Lee Crosby et al., "Ketogenic Diets and Chronic Disease: Weighing the Benefits Against the Risks," *Frontiers in Nutrition* (July 16, 2021), doi:10.3389/fnut.2021 .702802.

12. Josef Langfort et al., "Effect of Low-Carbohydrate-Ketogenic Diet on Metabolic and Hormonal Responses to Graded Exercise in Men," *Journal of Physiology and Pharmacology* 47, no. 2 (June 1996): 361–71, https://pubmed.ncbi.nlm.nih.gov/8807563/.

13. Christina Tsigalou et al., "Mediterranean Diet as a Tool to Combat Inflammation and Chronic Diseases. An Overview," *Biomedicines* 8, no. 7 (July 8, 2020), doi:10.3390 /biomedicines8070201; Kenia M. B. Carvalho et al., "Does the Mediterranean Diet Protect Against Stress-Induced Inflammatory Activation in European Adolescents? The HELENA Study," *Nutrients* 10, no. 11 (November 15, 2018): 1770, doi:10.3390 /nu10111770.

14. Eveline Deloose et al., "The Migrating Motor Complex: Control Mechanisms and Its Role in Health and Disease," *Nature Reviews Gastroenterology & Hepatology* 9 (March 27, 2012): 271–85, doi:10.1038/nrgastro.2012.57.

15. A. Zubrzycki et al., "The Role of Low-Calorie Diets and Intermittent Fasting in the Treatment of Obesity and Type-2 Diabetes," *Journal of Physiology and Pharmacology* 69, no. 5 (2018): 663–83, doi:10.26402/jpp.2018.5.02; Antonio Real-Hohn et al., "The Synergism of High-Intensity Intermittent Exercise and Every-Other-Day Intermittent Fasting Regimen on Energy Metabolism Adaptations Includes Hexokinase Activity and Mitochondrial Efficiency," *PLoS One* 13, no. 12 (December 21, 2018): e0202784, doi:10.1371/journal.pone.0202784.

16. Maarten R. Soeters et al., "Intermittent Fasting Does Not Affect Whole-Body Glucose, Lipid, or Protein Metabolism," *American Journal of Clinical Nutrition* 90, no. 5 (November 2009): 1244–51, doi:10.3945/ajcn.2008.27327.

17. Yuko Nakamura, Brian R. Walker, and Toshikazu Ikuta, "Systematic Review and Meta-Analysis Reveals Acutely Elevated Plasma Cortisol Following Fasting but Not Less Severe Calorie Restriction," *International Journal on the Biology of Stress* 19, no. 2 (November 19, 2015): 151–7, doi:10.3109/10253890.2015.1121984.

18. Giulia Salvadori, Mario Giuseppe Mirisola, and Valter D. Longo, "Intermittent and Periodic Fasting, Hormones, and Cancer Prevention," *Cancers* 13, no. 18 (September 13, 2021): 4587, doi:10.3390/cancers13184587.

19. Thomas Jensen et al., "Fructose and Sugar: A Major Mediator of Non-Alcoholic Fatty Liver Disease," *Journal of Hepatology* 68, no. 5 (May 1, 2018): 1063–75, doi:10.1016/j.jhep.2018.01.019.

20. William R. Lovallo et al., "Cortisol Responses to Mental Stress, Exercise, and Meals Following Caffeine Intake in Men and Women," *Pharmacology Biochemistry and Behavior* 83, no. 3 (March 2006):441–47, doi:10.1016/j.pbb.2006.03.005.

21. James H. O'Keefe et al., "Alcohol and Cardiovascular Health: The Dose Makes the Poison . . . or the Remedy," *Mayo Clinic Proceedings* 89, no. 3 (March 1, 2014): 382–93, doi:10.1016/j.mayocp.2013.11.005; Ning Xia et al., "Antioxidant Effects of Resveratrol in the Cardiovascular System," *British Journal of Pharmacology* 174, no. 12 (April 5, 2016): 1633–46, doi:10.1111/bph.13492.

22. Elodie Jean-Marie, Didier Bereau, and Jean-Charles Robinson, "Benefits of Polyphenols and Methylxanthines from Cocoa Beans on Dietary Metabolic Disorders," *Foods* 10, no. 9 (August 31, 2021): 2049, doi:10.3390/foods10092049.

23. Laura Maintz and Natalija Novak, "Histamine and Histamine Intolerance," *American Journal of Clinical Nutrition* 85, no. 5 (May 2007): 1185–96, doi:10.1093/ajcn/85.5.1185.

24. Janani Muthukumar et al., "Food and Food Products Associated with Food Allergy and Food Intolerance—An Overview," *Food Research International* 138, Part B (December 2020): 109780, doi:10.1016/j.foodres.2020.109780.

25. Kristin Schmidt et al., "Prebiotic Intake Reduces the Waking Cortisol Response and Alters Emotional Bias in Healthy Volunteers," *Psychopharmacology* 232 (December 3, 2014): 1793–1801, doi:10.1007/s00213-014-3810-0.

## Chapter 7

1. Marcella Balbo, Rachel Leproult, and Eve Van Cauter, "Impact of Sleep and Its Disturbances on Hypothalamo-Pituitary-Adrenal Axis Activity," *International Journal of Endocrinology* 2010 (June 9, 2010): 1–16, doi:10.1155/2010/759234.

2. Theresa M. Buckley and Alan F. Schatzberg, "On the Interactions of the Hypothalamic-Pituitary-Adrenal (HPA) Axis and Sleep: Normal HPA Axis Activity and Circadian Rhythm, Exemplary Sleep Disorders," *Journal of Clinical Endocrinology & Metabolism* 90, no. 5 (May 1, 2005): 3106–14, doi:10.1210/jc.2004-1056.

3. Michael Irwin et al., "Effects of Sleep and Sleep Deprivation on Catecholamine and Interleukin-2 Levels in Humans: Clinical Implications," *Journal of Clinical Endocrinology & Metabolism* 84, no. 6 (June 1, 1999): 1979–85, doi:10.1210/jcem.84.6.5788.

4. Alexandros N. Vgontzas et al., "Daytime Napping After a Night of Sleep Loss Decreases Sleepiness, Improves Performance, and Causes Beneficial Changes in Cortisol and Interleukin-6 Secretion," *American Journal of Physiology Endocrinology and Metabolism* 292, no. 1 (January 1, 2007): E253–61, doi:10.1152/ajpendo.00651.2005.

5. Russel J. Reiter et al., "Melatonin as an Antioxidant: Under Promises but Over Delivers," *Journal of Pineal Research* 61 no. 3 (October 2016): 253–78, doi:10.1111/jpi.12360.

6. Nadia Aalling Jessen et al., "The Glymphatic System: A Beginner's Guide," *Neurochemical Research* 40 (May 7, 2015): 2583–99, doi:10.1007/s11064-015-1581-6.

7. Bart van Alphen et al., "A Deep Sleep Stage in *Drosophila* with a Functional Role in Waste Clearance," *Science Advances* 7, no. 4 (2021), doi:10.1016/B978-0-12-822963-7.00037-2.

8. Christopher M. Depner, Ellen R. Stothard, and Kenneth P. Wright Jr., "Metabolic Consequences of Sleep and Circadian Disorders," *Macrovascular Complications in Diabetes* 14 (May 10, 2014): 507, doi:10.1007/s11892-014-0507-z.

9. Camila Hirotsu, Sergio Tufik, and Monica Levy Andersen, "Interactions Between Sleep, Stress, and Metabolism: From Physiological to Pathological Conditions," *Sleep Science* 8, no. 3 (November 2015): 143–52, doi:10.1016/j.slsci.2015.09.002.

10. Siegfried Wahl et al., "The Inner Clock—Blue Light Sets the Human Rhythm," *Journal of Biophotonics* (August 21, 2019), doi:10.1002/jbio.201900102.

11. Mariana G. Figueiro and Mark S. Rea, "The Effects of Red and Blue Lights on Circadian Variations in Cortisol, Alpha Amylase, and Melatonin," *International Journal of Endocrinology* 2010 (June 24, 2010): 1–9, doi:10.1155/2010/829351.

12. Angela Smith Lillehei et al., "Effect of Inhaled Lavender and Sleep Hygiene on Self-Reported Sleep Issues: A Randomized Controlled Trial," *Journal of Alternative and Complementary Medicine* 21, no. 7 (July 2, 2015): 430–8, doi:10.1089/acm.2014.0327.

13. Giulia Lara Poerio et al., "More Than a Feeling: Autonomous Sensory Meridian Response (ASMR) Is Characterized by Reliable Changes in Affect and Physiology," *PLoS One* 13, no. 6 (June 20, 2018): e0196645, doi:10.1371/journal.pone.0196645.

14. Malka N. Halgamuge, "Critical Time Delay of the Pineal Melatonin Rhythm in Humans Due to Weak Electromagnetic Exposure," *Indian Journal of Biochemistry & Biophysics* 50, no. 4 (August 2013): 259–65, https://pubmed.ncbi.nlm.nih.gov/24772943/.

15. Shahab Haghayegh et al., "Before-Bedtime Passive Body Heating by Warm Shower or Bath to Improve Sleep: A Systematic Review and Meta-Analysis," *Sleep Medicine Reviews* 46 (August 2019): 124–35, doi:10.1016/j.smrv.2019.04.008.

16. Stella Iacovides and Rebecca M. Meiring, "The Effect of a Ketogenic Diet Versus a High-Carbohydrate, Low-Fat Diet on Sleep, Cognition, Thyroid Function, and Cardiovascular Health Independent of Weight Loss: Study Protocol for a Randomized Controlled Trial," *Trials* 19, no. 1 (January 23, 2018): 62, doi:10.1186/s13063-018-2462-5.

17. Leah A. Irish et al., "The Role of Sleep Hygiene in Promoting Public Health: A Review of Empirical Evidence," *Sleep Medicine Reviews* 22 (August 2015): 23–36, doi:10.1016/j.smrv.2014.10.001.

18. Andrew Herxheimer and Keith J. Petrie, "Melatonin for the prevention and treatment of jet lag," Cochrane Database of Systematic Reviews 2 (2002): CD001520, doi:10.1002/14651858.CD001520.

19. Josef Fritz et al., "A Chronobiological Evaluation of the Acute Effects of Daylight Saving Time on Traffic Accident Risk," *Current Biology* 30, no. 4 (2020): 729–32, doi:10.1016/j.cub.2019.12.045.

## Chapter 8

1. Pedro Mateos-Aparicio and Antonio Rodríguez-Moreno, "The Impact of Studying Brain Plasticity," *Frontiers in Cellular Neuroscience* (February 27, 2019), doi:10.3389/fncel.2019.00066.

2. Rollin McCraty and Doc Childre, "The Grateful Heart: The Psychophysiology of Appreciation," in *The Psychology of Gratitude*, ed. Robert A. Emmons and Michael E. McCullough (Oxford: Oxford University Press, 2004): 230–55; Marta Jackowska et al., "The Impact of a Brief Gratitude Intervention on Subjective Well-Being, Biology and Sleep," *Journal of Health Psychology* 21, no. 10 (2016): 2207–17, doi:10.1177/1359105315572455; Alison Killen and Ann Macaskill, "Using a Gratitude Intervention to Enhance Well-Being in Older Adults," *Journal of Happiness Studies* 16 (2015): 947–64, doi:10.1007/s10902-014-9542-3; Sheung-Tak Cheng, Pui Ki Tsui, and John H. M. Lam, "Improving Mental Health in Health Care Practitioners: Randomized Controlled Trial of a Gratitude Intervention," *Journal of Consulting and Clinical Psychology* 83, no. 1 (February 2015): 177–186, doi:10.1037/a0037895.

3. Prathik Kini et al., "The Effects of Gratitude Expression on Neural Activity," *Neuroimage* 128 (2016): 1–10, doi:10.1016/j.neuroimage.2015.12.040.

4. Sara B. Algoe and Baldwin M. Way, "Evidence for a Role of the Oxytocin System, Indexed by Genetic Variation in *CD38*, in the Social Bonding Effects of Expressed Gratitude," Social Cognitive and Affective Neuroscience 9, no. 12 (2014): 1855–61, doi:10.1093/scan/nst182.

5. Seoyoung Yoon and Yong-Ku Kim, "The Role of the Oxytocin System in Anxiety Disorders," in *Anxiety Disorders, Advances in Experimental Medicine and Biology, vol. 1191*, ed. Yong-Yu Kim (The Gateway, Singapore: Springer Nature, 2020), doi:10.1007/978-981-32-9705-0_7; R. J. Windle et al., "Central Oxytocin Administration Reduces Stress-Induced Corticosterone Release and Anxiety Behavior in Rats," *Endocrinology* 138, no. 7 (1997): 2829–34, doi:10.1210/endo.138.7.5255; Burel R. Goodin, Timothy J. Ness, and Meredith T. Robbins, "Oxytocin—A Multifunctional Analgesic for Chronic Deep Tissue Pain," *Current Pharmaceutical Design* 21, no. 7 (2015): 906–13, doi:10.2174/1381612820666141027111843; Haiying Shao and Ming-Sheng Zhou, "Cardiovascular Action of Oxytocin," *Journal of Autacoids and Hormones* 3 (2014): e124, doi:10.4172/2161-0479.1000e124.

6. J. Gutkowska et al., "Oxytocin Is a Cardiovascular Hormone," *Brazilian Journal of Medical and Biological Research* 33, no. 6 (2000): 625–33, doi:10.1590/S0100-879X2000000600003.

7. Luciano Bernardi, Camillo Porta, and Peter Sleight, "Cardiovascular, Cerebrovascular, and Respiratory Changes Induced by Different Types of Music in Musicians

and Non-Musicians: The Importance of Silence," *Heart* 92, no. 4 (March 14, 2006): 445–52, doi:10.1136/hrt.2005.064600; Imke Kirste et al., "Is Silence Golden? Effects of Auditory Stimuli and Their Absence on Adult Hippocampal Neurogenesis," *Brain Structure and Function* 220, no. 2 (December 1, 2013):1221–28, doi:10.1007/s00429-013-0679-3.

8. Jim Lagopoulos et al., "Increased Theta and Alpha EEG Activity During Nondirective Meditation," *Journal of Alternative and Complementary Medicine* 15, no. 11 (2009): 1187–92, doi:10.1089/acm.2009.0113.

9. Richard J. Davidson and Antoine Lutz, "Buddha's Brain: Neuroplasticity and Meditation [In the Spotlight]," *IEEE Signal Processing Magazine* 25, no. 1 (2008): 176, doi:10.1109/MSP.2008.4431873.

10. Linda E. Carlson et al., "Mindfulness-Based Stress Reduction in Relation to Quality of Life, Mood, Symptoms of Stress and Levels of Cortisol, Dehydroepiandrosterone Sulfate (DHEAS) and Melatonin in Breast and Prostate Cancer Outpatients," *Psychoneuroendocrinology* 29, no. 4 (May 2004): 448–74, doi:10.1016/s0306-4530(03)00054-4; Adam Koncz, Zsolt Demetrovics, and Zsofia K. Takacs, "Meditation Interventions Efficiently Reduce Cortisol Levels of At-Risk Samples: A Meta-Analysis," *Health Psychology Review* 1, no. 15 (July 7, 2020): 56–84, doi:10.1080/17437199.2020.1760727; Richard Bränström, Pia Kvillemo, and Torbjörn Akerstedt, "Effects of Mindfulness Training on Levels of Cortisol in Cancer Patients," *Psychosomatics* 54, no. 2 (2013): 158–64, doi:10.1016/j.psym.2012.04.007.

11. Therese J. Borchard, "Spirituality and Prayer Relieve Stress," PsychCentral, March 21, 2010, https://psychcentral.com/blog/spirituality-and-prayer-relieve-stress.

12. Lorena Angela Cattaneo et al., "Is Low Heart Rate Variability Associated with Emotional Dysregulation, Psychopathological Dimensions, and Prefrontal Dysfunctions? An Integrative View," *Journal of Personalized Medicine* 11, no. 9 (2021): 872, doi:10.3390/jpm11090872.

13. B. Bonaz, V. Sinniger, and S. Pellissier, "Vagal Tone: Effects on Sensitivity, Motility, and Inflammation," *Neurogastroenterology & Motility* 28, no. 4 (2016): 455–62, doi:10.1111/nmo.12817.

14. Angele McGrady et al., "Effect of Biofeedback-Assisted Relaxation on Blood Pressure and Cortisol Levels in Normotensives and Hypertensives," *Journal of Behavioral Medicine* 10, no. 3 (June 1987): 301–10. doi:10.1007/bf00846543; Yuka Kotozaki et al., "Biofeedback-Based Training for Stress Management in Daily Hassles: An Intervention Study," *Brain and Behavior* 4, no. 4 (July 2014): 566–79. doi:10.1002/brb3.241.

15. V. Doreen Wagner, Sharon M. Pearcey, and G. Karakayali, "141. Perceived Stress and Salivary Cortisol in Educators: Comparison Among Three Stress Reduction Activities," *Brain, Behavior, and Immunity* 40, Supplement (September 2014): e41, doi:10.1016/j.bbi.2014.06.161; Jeremy West et al., "Effects of Hatha Yoga and African Dance on Perceived Stress, Affect, and Salivary Cortisol," *Annals of Behavioral Medicine,* 28, no. 2 (October 2004): 114–18, doi:10.1207/s15324796abm2802_6.

16. Adnan I. Qureshi et al., "Cat Ownership and the Risk of Fatal Cardiovascular Diseases. Results from the Second National Health and Nutrition Examination Study Mortality Follow-up Study," *Journal of Vascular and Interventional Neurology* 2, no. 1 (2009): 132–5, https://www.ncbi.nlm.nih.gov/pmc/articles/PMC3317329/.

17. Karen Allen, Barbara E. Shykoff, and Joseph L. Izzo Jr, "Pet Ownership, but Not ACE Inhibitor Therapy, Blunts Home Blood Pressure Responses to Mental Stress," *Hypertension* 38, no. 4 (October 2001): 815–20, doi:10.1161/hyp.38.4.815; Andrea

Beetz et al., "Psychosocial and Psychophysiological Effects of Human-Animal Inter-actions: The Possible Role of Oxytocin," *Frontiers in Psychology* 3 (July 9, 2012), doi:10.3389/fpsyg.2012.00234.

18. MaryCarol R. Hunter, Brenda W. Gillespie, and Sophie Y.-P. Chen, "Urban Nature Experiences Reduce Stress in the Context of Daily Life Based on Salivary Biomark-ers," *Frontiers in Psychology* 10 (April 4, 2019), doi:10.3389/fpsyg.2019.00722.

19. Qing Li, "Effect of Forest Bathing Trips on Human Immune Function," *Environmen-tal Health and Preventative Medicine* 15 (2010): 9–17, doi:10.1007/s12199-008-0068-3.

20. Margaret M. Hansen, Reo Jones, and Kirsten Tocchini, "Shinrin-Yoku (Forest Bathing) and Nature Therapy: A State-of-the-Art Review," *International Journal of Environmental Research and Public Health* 14, no. 8 (2017): 851, doi:10.3390/ijerph 14080851.

21. Bonaz, Sinniger, and Pellissier, "Vagal Tone"; R. Passi et al., "Electrical Ground-ing Improves Vagal Tone in Preterm Infants," *Neonatology* 112 (2017): 187–92, doi:10.1159/000475744.

22. Sigrid Breit et al., "Vagus Nerve as Modulator of the Brain–Gut Axis in Psychi-atric and Inflammatory Disorders," *Frontiers in Psychiatry* (2018), doi:10.3389/fpsyt .2018.00044.

23. Valentin A. Pavlov and Kevin J. Tracey, "The Vagus Nerve and the Inflammatory Reflex—Linking Immunity and Metabolism," *Nature Reviews Endocrinology* 8 (2012): 743–54, doi:10.1038/nrendo.2012.189.

24. James Oschman, Gaetan Chevalier, and Richard Brown, "The Effects of Grounding (Earthing) on Inflammation, the Immune Response, Wound Healing, and Preven-tion and Treatment of Chronic Inflammatory and Autoimmune Diseases," *Journal of Inflammation Research* 8 (2015): 83–96, doi:10.2147/JIR.S69656.

25. Min-sun Lee et al., "Interaction with Indoor Plants May Reduce Psychological and Physiological Stress by Suppressing Autonomic Nervous System Activity in Young Adults: A Randomized Crossover Study," *Journal of Physiosocial Anthropology* 34 (2015): 21, doi:10.1186/s40101-015-0060-8.

26. Agnes E. Van Den Berg and Mariëtte H. G. Custers, "Gardening Promotes Neuro-endocrine and Affective Restoration from Stress," *Journal of Health Psychology* 16, no. 1 (June 3, 2010): 3–11, doi:10.1177/1359105310365577.

27. Lee S. Berk et al., "Neuroendocrine and Stress Hormone Changes During Mirth-ful Laughter," *American Journal of the Medical Sciences* 298, no. 6 (1989): 390–6, doi:10.1097/00000441-198912000-00006.

28. Michael Miller and William F. Fry, "The Effect of Mirthful Laughter on the Human Cardiovascular System," *Medical Hypotheses* 73, no. 5 (2009): 636–9, doi:10.1016/j .mehy.2009.02.044; JongEun Yim, "Therapeutic Benefits of Laughter in Mental Health: A Theoretical Review," *Tohoku Journal of Experimental Medicine* 239, no. 3 (2016): 243–9, doi:10.1620/tjem.239.243.

29. Yuuki Ooishi et al., "Increase in Salivary Oxytocin and Decrease in Salivary Cortisol After Listening to Relaxing Slow-Tempo and Exciting Fast-Tempo Music," *PLOS ONE* 12, no. 12 (December 6, 2017): e0189075, doi:10.1371/journal.pone.0189075.

30. Daniel Leubner and Thilo Hinterberger, "Reviewing the Effectiveness of Music Interventions in Treating Depression," *Frontiers in Psychology* (2017), doi:10.3389 /fpsyg.2017.01109.

31. Diletta Calamassi and Gian Paolo Pomponi, "Music Tuned to 440 Hz Versus 432 Hz and the Health Effects: A Double-Blind Cross-Over Pilot Study," *Explore (NY)* 15,

no. 4 (2019): 283–90, doi:10.1016/j.explore.2019.04.001; Kaho Akimoto et al., "Effect of 528 Hz Music on the Endocrine System and Autonomic Nervous System," *Health* 10, no. 9 (2018): 1159–70, doi:10.4236/health.2018.109088.

32. Leila Chaieb et al., "Auditory Beat Stimulation and Its Effects on Cognition and Mood States," *Frontiers in Psychiatry* (2015), doi:10.3389/fpsyt.2015.00070.

33. S. W. Porges, "Orienting in a Defensive World: Mammalian Modifications of Our Evolutionary Heritage. A Polyvagal Theory," *Psychophysiology* 32, no. 4 (1995): 301–18, doi:10.1111/j.1469-8986.1995.tb01213.x.

34. Robert J. Ellis and Julian F. Thayer, "Music and Autonomic Nervous System (Dys)Function," *Music Perception* 27, no. 4 (2010): 317–26, doi:10.1525/mp.2010 .27.4.317.

35. West et al., "Effects of Hatha Yoga and African Dance on Perceived Stress, Affect, and Salivary Cortisol."

36. Young-Ja Jeong et al., "Dance Movement Therapy Improves Emotional Responses and Modulates Neurohormones in Adolescents with Mild Depression," *International Journal of Neuroscience* 115, no. 12 (2009): 1711–20, doi:10.1080/00207450590958574; Jacqueline C. Dominguez et al., "Improving Cognition Through Dance in Older Filipinos with Mild Cognitive Impairment," *Current Alzheimer Research* 15, no. 12 (2018): 1136–41, doi:10.2174/1567205015666180801112428.

37. M. L. Hannuksela and S. Ellahham, "Benefits and Risks of Sauna Bathing," *American Journal of Medicine* 110, no. 2 (February 1, 2001): 118–26, doi:10.1016/s0002 -9343(00)00671-9; Katriina Kukkonen-Harjula et al., "Haemodynamic and Hormonal Responses to Heat Exposure in a Finnish Sauna Bath," *European Journal of Applied Physiology and Occupational Physiology* 58, no. 5 (March 1989): 543–50, doi:10.1007/bf02330710; Timo Laatikainen et al., "Response of Plasma Endorphins, Prolactin and Catecholamines in Women to Intense Heat in a Sauna," *European Journal of Applied Physiology and Occupational Physiology* 57, no. 1 (January 1988): 98–102, doi:10.1007/bf00691246.

38. Mary H. Burleson, Wenda R. Trevathan, and Michael Todd, "In the Mood for Love or Vice Versa? Exploring the Relations Among Sexual Activity, Physical Affection, Affect, and Stress in the Daily Lives of Mid-Aged Women," *Archives of Sexual Behavior* 36, no. 3 (November 16, 2006): 357–68, doi:10.1007/s10508-006-9071-1.

39. Kathleen C. Light, Karen M. Grewen, and Janet A. Amico, "More Frequent Partner Hugs and Higher Oxytocin Levels Are Linked to Lower Blood Pressure and Heart Rate in Premenopausal Women," *Biological Psychology* 69, no. 1 (2005): 5–21, doi:10.1016/j.biopsycho.2004.11.002.

40. Navneet Magon and Sanjay Kalra, "The Orgasmic History of Oxytocin: Love, Lust, and Labor," *Indian Journal of Endocrinology and Metabolism* 15 supplement 3 (2011): S156–61, doi:10.4103/2230-8210.84851.

41. Susan A. Hall et al., "Sexual Activity, Erectile Dysfunction, and Incident Cardiovascular Events," *Preventive Cardiology* 105, no. 2 (2010): 192–97, doi:10.1016/j.am jcard.2009.08.671.

42. George Davey Smith, Stephen Frankel, and John Yarnell, "Sex and Death: Are They Related? Findings from the Caerphilly Cohort Study," *BMJ* 315 (1997): 1641, doi:10.1136/bmj.315.7123.1641.

43. Hayley Wright and Rebecca A. Jenks, "Sex on the Brain! Associations Between Sexual Activity and Cognitive Function in Older Age," *Age and Ageing* 45, no. 2 (2016): 313–17, doi:10.1093/ageing/afv197.

44. Leslie J. Seltzer, Toni E. Ziegler and Seth D. Pollak, "Social Vocalizations Can Release Oxytocin in Humans," *Proceedings of the Royal Society B Biological Sciences* 277 (2010): 2661–66, doi:10.1098/rspb.2010.0567.

45. Joshua M. Smyth et al., "Online Positive Affect Journaling in the Improvement of Mental Distress and Well-Being in General Medical Patients with Elevated Anxiety Symptoms: A Preliminary Randomized Controlled Trial," *JMIR Mental Health* 5, no. 4 (October–December 2018): E11290, doi:10.2196/11290; James W. Pennebaker, "Expressive Writing in Psychological Science," *Perspectives on Psychological Science* 13, no. 2 (2018): 226–29, doi:10.1177/1745691617707315.

46. Joan I. Rosenberg, *90 Seconds to a Life You Love: How to Master Your Difficult Feelings to Cultivate Lasting Confidence, Resilience, and Authenticity* (New York: Little, Brown, 2019).

47. Sara Sahranavard et al., "The Effectiveness of Stress-Management-Based Cognitive-Behavioral Treatments on Anxiety Sensitivity, Positive and Negative Affect and Hope," *BioMedicine* 8, no. 4 (2018): 23, doi:10.1051/bmdcn/2018080423.

48. Francine Shapiro, "The Role of Eye Movement Desensitization and Reprocessing (EMDR) Therapy in Medicine: Addressing the Psychological and Physical Symptoms Stemming from Adverse Life Experience," *Permanente Journal* 18, no. 1 (2014): 71–77, doi:10.7812/TPP/13-098.

49. Lia Naor and Ofra Mayseless, "The Wilderness Solo Experience: A Unique Practice of Silence and Solitude for Personal Growth," *Frontiers in Psychology* 11 (2020):547067, doi:10.3389/fpsyg.2020.547067; Micaela Rodriguez, Benjamin W. Bellet, and Richard J. McNally, "Reframing Time Spent Alone: Reappraisal Buffers the Emotional Effects of Isolation," *Cognitive Therapy and Research* 44 (2020):1–16, doi:10.1007/s10608-020-10128-x.

50. Hui-Chen Lu and Ken Mackie, "An Introduction to the Endogenous Cannabinoid System," *Biological Psychiatry* 79, no. 7 (2016): 516–25, doi:10.1016/j.biopsych.2015.07.028.

51. University of Illinois at Chicago, "Low-Dose THC Can Relieve Stress; More Does Just the Opposite," ScienceDaily, June 2, 2017, https://www.sciencedaily.com/releases/2017/06/170602155252.htm.

52. Nathalie Niederhoffer et al., "Effects of Cannabinoids on Adrenaline Release from Adrenal Medullary Cells," *British Journal of Pharmacology* 134, no. 6 (January 29, 2009): 1319–27, doi:10.1038/sj.bjp.0704359; Anita Cservenka, Sarah Lahanas, and Julieanne Dotson-Bossert, "Marijuana Use and Hypothalamic-Pituitary-Adrenal Axis Functioning in Humans," *Frontiers in Psychiatry* 9 (October 1, 2018), doi:10.3389/fpsyt.2018.00472; Mohini Ranganathan et al., "The Effects of Cannabinoids on Serum Cortisol and Prolactin in Humans," *Psychopharmacology* 203, no. 4 (December 16, 2008): 737–44, doi:10.1007/s00213-008-1422-2.

53. Kevin M Swiatek, Kim Jordan, and Julie Coffman, "New Use for an Old Drug: Oral Ketamine for Treatment-Resistant Depression," *BMJ Case Reports* 2016 (2016): bcr2016216088, doi:10.1136/bcr-2016-216088; Mark T. Wagner et al., "Therapeutic Effect of Increased Openness: Investigating Mechanism of Action in MDMA-Assisted Psychotherapy," *Journal of Psychopharmacology* 31, no. 8 (2018): 967–74, doi:10.1177/0269881117711712; Roland R. Griffiths et al., "Psilocybin Produces Substantial and Sustained Decreases in Depression and Anxiety in Patients with Life-Threatening Cancer: A Randomized Double-Blind Trial," *Journal of*

*Psychopharmacology* 30, no. 12 (2016): 1181–97, doi:10.1177/0269881116675513; Jerome Sarris et al., "Ayahuasca Use and Reported Effects on Depression and Anxiety Symptoms: An International Cross-Sectional Study of 11,912 Consumers," *Journal of Affective Disorders Reports* 4 (2021): 100098, doi:10.1016/j.jadr.2021.100098; Fernanda Palhano-Fontes et al., "Rapid Antidepressant Effects of the Psychedelic Ayahuasca in Treatment-Resistant Depression: A Randomized Placebo-Controlled Trial," *Psychological Medicine* 49, no. 4 (2019): 655–63, doi:10.1017/S0033291718001356.

54. Liana Fattore et al., "Psychedelics and reconsolidation of traumatic and appetitive maladaptive memories: focus on cannabinoids and ketamine," *Psychopharmacology* 235 (2018): 433–45, doi:10.1007/s00213-017-4793-4.

55. R. L. Carhart-Harris et al., "Psychedelics and Connectedness," *Psychopharmacology* 235 (2018): 547–50, doi:10.1007/s00213-017-4701-y.

56. Ira Byock, "Taking Psychedelics Seriously," *Journal of Palliative Medicine* 21, no. 4 (2018): 417–21, doi:10.1089/jpm.2017.0684.

57. Rafael G. dos Santos et al., "Antidepressive and Anxiolytic Effects of Ayahuasca: A Systematic Literature Review of Animal and Human Studies," *Brazilian Journal of Psychiatry* 38, no. 1 (2016): 65–72, doi:10.1590/1516-4446-2015-1701; Daniel F. Jiménez-Garrido et al., "Effects of Ayahuasca on Mental Health and Quality of Life in Naïve Users: A Longitudinal and Cross-Sectional Study Combination," *Scientific Reports* 10 (2020): 4075, doi:10.1038/s41598-020-61169-x.

58. V. Kh. Khavinson and V. N. Anisimov, "Peptide Regulation of Aging: 35-Year Research Experience," *Biogerontology* 148 (2009): 94, doi: 10.1007/s10517-009-0650-8.

59. Chun-Yan Shen et al., "Anti-ageing active ingredients from herbs and nutraceuticals used in traditional Chinese medicine: pharmacological mechanisms and implications for drug discovery," *British Journal of Pharmacology* 174, no. 11 (2017): 1395–1425, doi:10.1111/bph.13631.

60. Mandana Bagherian, Adis Keraskian Mojembari, and Mohammad Hakami, "The Effects of Homeopathic Medicines on Reducing the Symptoms of Anxiety and Depression: Randomized, Double Blind and Placebo Controlled," *Journal of Traditional Medicine & Clinical Naturopathy* 3 (2014): 167, doi: 10.4172/2167-1206.1000167; Babar Ali et al., "Essential oils used in aromatherapy: A systemic review," *Asian Pacific Journal of Tropical Biomedicine* 5, no. 8 (2015): 601–11, doi:10.1016/j.apjtb.2015.05.007; Donna Bach et al., "Clinical EFT (Emotional Freedom Techniques) Improves Multiple Physiological Markers of Health," *Journal of Evidence-Based Integrative Medicine* 24 (2019): 2515690X18823691, doi:10.1177/2515690X18823691; Fateme Nazari, Mojtaba Mirzamohamadi, and Hojatollah Yousefi, "The effect of massage therapy on occupational stress of Intensive Care Unit nurses," *Iranian Journal of Nursing and Midwifery Research* 20, no. 4 (2015): 508–15, doi:10.4103/1735-9066.161001; Kristen Sparrow and Brenda Golianu, "Does Acupuncture Reduce Stress Over Time? A Clinical Heart Rate Variability Study in Hypertensive Patients," *Medical Acupuncture* 26, no. 5 (2014): 286–94, doi:10.1089/acu.2014.1050.

61. Maria Meier et al., "Standardized massage interventions as protocols for the induction of psychophysiological relaxation in the laboratory: a block randomized, controlled trial," *Scientific Reports* 10 (2020): 14774, doi:10.1038/s41598-020-71173-w; David E. McManus, "Reiki Is Better Than Placebo and Has Broad Potential as a Complementary Health Therapy," *Journal of Evidence-Based Integrative Medicine* (2017): 1051-7, doi:10.1177/2156587217728644.

# Chapter 9

1. Ulrike Rimmele et al., "Trained Men Show Lower Cortisol, Heart Rate and Psychological Responses to Psychosocial Stress Compared with Untrained Men," *Psychoneuroendocrinology* 32, no. 6 (July 2007): 627–35, doi:10.1016/j.psyneuen.2007.04.005.
2. Wilfried Kindermann et al., "Catecholamines, Growth Hormone, Cortisol, Insulin, and Sex Hormones in Anaerobic and Aerobic Exercise," *European Journal of Applied Physiology and Occupational Physiology* 49, no. 3 (September 1982): 389–99, doi:10.1007/bf00441300; Jennifer L. J. Heaney et al., "Preliminary Evidence That Exercise Dependence Is Associated with Blunted Cardiac and Cortisol Reactions to Acute Psychological Stress," *International Journal of Psychophysiology* 79, no. 2 (February 2011): 323–29, doi:10.1016/j.ijpsycho.2010.11.010.
3. Matteo Bonato et al., "Salivary cortisol concentration after high-intensity interval exercise: Time of day and chronotype effect," *Chronobiology International* 34, no. 6 (April 2017): 698–707, doi:10.1080/07420528.2017.1311336.
4. Lauren L. Drogos et al., "Aerobic Exercise Increases Cortisol Awakening Response in Older Adults," *Psychoneuroendocrinology* 103 (May 2019): 241–48, doi:10.1016/j.psyneuen.2019.01.012.
5. E. E. Hill et al., "Exercise and circulating cortisol levels: The intensity threshold effect," *Journal of Endocrinological Investigation* 31 (2008): 587–91, doi:10.1007/BF03345606.
6. Alsayed A. Shanb and Enas F. Youseff, "The impact of adding weight-bearing exercise versus nonweight bearing programs to the medical treatment of elderly patients with osteoporosis," *Journal of Family and Community Medicine* 21, no. 3 (2014): 176–81, doi:10.4103/2230-8229.142972.
7. Rachel Dermack, "Long-Distance Running: An Investigation Into Its Impact on Human Health," *People, Ideas, and Things (PIT) Journal* 6 (2015).
8. Elizabeth M. Jenkins et al., "Do Stair Climbing Exercise 'Snacks' Improve Cardiorespiratory Fitness?", *Applied Physiology, Nutrition, and Metabolism* (January 2019), doi:10.1139/apnm-2018-0675.
9. Phil Page, "Current concepts in muscle stretching for exercise and rehabilitation," *International Journal of Sports Physical Therapy* 7, no. 1 (February 2012): 109–19.
10. Catherine Woodyard, "Exploring the therapeutic effects of yoga and its ability to increase quality of life," *International Journal of Yoga* 4, no. 2 (2011): 49–64, doi:10.4103/0973-6131.85485.
11. June Kloubec, "Pilates: how to does it work and who needs it?", *Muscles, Ligaments and Tendons Journal* 1, no. 2 (2011): 61–6.
12. Styliani Douka, et al., "Traditional Dance Improves the Physical Fitness and Well-Being of the Elderly," *Frontiers in Aging Neuroscience* (April 2019), doi:10.3389/fnagi.2019.00075.
13. Pei-Shiun Chang et al., "Physical and Psychological Health Outcomes of Qigong Exercise in Older Adults: A Systematic Review and Meta-Analysis," *American Journal of Chinese Medicine* 47, no. 2 (2019): 301–22, doi:10.1142/S0192415X19500149; Angus P. Yu et al., "Revealing the Neural Mechanisms Underlying the Beneficial Effects of Tai Chi: A Neuroimaging Perspective," *American Journal of Chinese Medicine* 46, no, 2 (2018): 231–59, doi:10.1142/S0192415X18500131.
14. Stuart M. Phillips and Richard A. Winett, "Uncomplicated resistance training and health-related outcomes: evidence for a public health mandate," *Current Sports Medicine Reports* 9, no. 4 (2010): 208–13, doi:10.1249/JSR.0b013e3181e7da73.

# Chapter 10

1. Shaheen E. Lakhan and Karen F. Vieira, "Nutritional therapies for mental disorders," *Nutrition Journal* 7 (2008): 2, doi:10.1186/1475-2891-7-2.

2. Suhyeon Kim et al., "GABA and l-theanine mixture decreases sleep latency and improves NREM sleep," *Pharmaceutical Biology* 59, no. 1 (2019): 64–72, doi:10.1080/13880209.2018.1557698.

3. Piril Hepsomali et al., "Effects of Oral Gamma-Aminobutyric Acid (GABA) Administration on Stress and Sleep in Humans: A Systematic Review," *Frontiers in Neuroscience* (2020), doi:10.3389/fnins.2020.00923.

4. Massimo E. Maffei, "5-Hydroxytryptophan (5-HTP): Natural Occurrence, Analysis, Biosynthesis, Biotechnology, Physiology and Toxicology," *International Journal of Molecular Sciences* 22, no. 1 (2021), doi:10.3390/ijms22010181.

5. Michael A. Starks et al., "The effects of phosphatidylserine on endocrine response to moderate intensity exercise," *Journal of the International Society of Sports Nutrition* 5, no. 11 (2008), doi:10.1186/1550-2783-5-11.

6. Adrian L. Lopresti et al., "An Investigation into the Stress-Relieving and Pharmacological Actions of an Ashwagandha (*Withania somnifera*) Extract," *Medicine* 98, no. 37 (September 2019): e17186, doi:10.1097/md.0000000000017186; K. Chandrasekhar, Jyoti Kapoor, and Sridhar Anishetty, "A prospective, randomized double-blind, placebo-controlled study of safety and efficacy of a high-concentration full-spectrum extract of ashwagandha root in reducing stress and anxiety in adults," *Indian Journal of Psychological Medicine* 34, no. 3 (July 2012): 255–62, doi:10.4103/0253-7176.106022; Jaysing Salve et al., "Adaptogenic and Anxiolytic Effects of Ashwagandha Root Extract in Healthy Adults: A Double-Blind, Randomized, Placebo-Controlled Clinical Study," *Cureus* 11, no. 12 (2019): e6466, doi:10.7759/cureus.6466.

7. Shawn M. Talbott, Julie A. Talbott, and Mike Pugh, "Effect of *Magnolia officinalis* and *Phellodendron amurense* (Relora®) on Cortisol and Psychological Mood State in Moderately Stressed Subjects," *Journal of the International Society of Sports Nutrition* 10, no. 1 (August 7, 2013), doi:10.1186/1550-2783-10-37; Catherine Ulbricht et al., "Banaba (Lagerstroemia speciosa L.): an evidence-based systematic review by the Natural Standard research collaboration," *Journal of Herbal Pharmacotherapy* 7, no. 1 (2007): 99–113.

8. Erik M. G. Olsson, Bo von Schéele, and Alexander G. Panossian, "A Randomised, Double-Blind, Placebo-Controlled, Parallel-Group Study of the Standardised Extract SHR-5 of the Roots of *Rhodiola rosea* in the Treatment of Subjects with Stress-Related Fatigue," *Planta Medica* 75, no. 2 (2009): 105–12, doi:10.1055/s-0028-1088346.

9. Marta Stachowicz and Anna Lebiedzińska, "The Effect of Diet Components on the Level of Cortisol," *European Food Research and Technology* 242, no. 12 (September 3, 2016): 2001–9, doi:10.1007/s00217-016-2772-3; Magdalena D. Cuciureanu and Robert Vink, "Magnesium and Stress," in *Magnesium in the Central Nervous System*, ed. R. Vink and M. Nechifor (Adelaide [AU]: University of Adelaide Press, 2011), https://www.ncbi.nlm.nih.gov/books/NBK507250/.

10. David O. Kennedy, "B Vitamins and the Brain: Mechanisms, Dose and Efficacy—A Review," *Nutrients* 8, no. 2 (2016): 68, doi:10.3390/nu8020068.

11. Shanshan Kong, Yanhui H. Zhang, and Weiqiang Zhang, "Regulation of Intestinal Epithelial Cells Properties and Functions by Amino Acids," *BioMed Research International* (May 2018), doi:10.1155/2018/2819154.

12. Kong, Zhang, and Zhang, "Regulation of Intestinal Epithelial Cells."

13. Giulia Pastorino et al., "Liquorice (*Glycyrrhiza glabra*): A phytochemical and phar-macological review," *Phytotherapy Research* 32, no. 12 (2018): 2323–39, doi:10.1002/ptr.6178; Thu Han Le Phan et al., "The Role of Processed *Aloe vera* Gel in Intestinal Tight Junction: An In Vivo and In Vitro Study," *International Journal of Molecular Sciences* 22, no. 12 (June 2021): 6515, doi:10.3390/ijms22126515.

## Chapter 11

1. Jing Du et al., "The Role of Nutrients in Protecting Mitochondrial Function and Neurotransmitter Signaling: Implications for the Treatment of Depression, PTSD, and Suicidal Behaviors," *Critical Reviews in Food Science and Nutrition* 56, no. 15 (2016), 2560–78, doi:10.1080/10408398.2013.876960.
2. Shankar Mondal, Bijay Ranjan Mirdha, and Sushil Chandra Mahapatra, "The Science Behind Sacredness of Tulsi (*Ocimum sanctum* Linn.)," *Indian Journal of Physiology and Pharmacology* 53, no. 4 (October 2009): 291–306, https://www.researchgate.net/publication/44636849_The_science_behind_sacredness_of_Tulsi_Ocimum_sanctum_Linn; Ben T. Gaffney, Helmut M. Hügel, and Peter A. Rich, "The Effects of *Eleutherococcus senticosus* and *Panax ginseng* on Steroidal Hormone Indices of Stress and Lymphocyte Subset Numbers in Endurance Athletes," *Life Sciences* 70, no. 4 (December 14, 2001): 431–42, doi:10.1016/s0024-3205(01)01394-7.
3. R. A. Isbrucker and George A. Burdock, "Risk and Safety Assessment on the Consumption of Licorice Root (*Glycyrrhiza* sp.), Its Extract and Powder as a Food Ingredient, with Emphasis on the Pharmacology and Toxicology of Glycyrrhizin," *Regulatory Toxicology and Pharmacology* 46, no. 3 (December 2006): 167–92, doi:10.1016/j.yrtph.2006.06.002.
4. J. Philip Karl et al., "Effects of Psychological, Environmental and Physical Stressors on the Gut Microbiota," *Frontiers in Microbiology* (2018), doi:10.3389/fmicb.2018.02013.
5. Javad Sharifi-Rad et al., "Probiotics: Versatile Bioactive Components in Promoting Human Health," *Medicina (Kaunas)* 56, no. 9 (August 2020): 433, doi:10.3390/medicina56090433.
6. Health Quality Ontario, "Fecal Microbiota Therapy for Clostridium difficile Infection: A Health Technology Assessment," *Ontario Health Technology Assessment Series* 16, no. 17 (July 2016): 1–69.
7. Susan Mills et al., "Precision Nutrition and the Microbiome, Part I: Current State of the Science," *Nutrients* 11, no. 4 (April 2019): 923, doi:10.3390/nu11040923.
8. Mathilde Versini et al., "Unraveling the Hygiene Hypothesis of helminthes and autoimmunity: origins, pathophysiology, and clinical applications," *BMC Medicine* 13 (April 2015), doi:10.1186/s12916-015-0306-7.
9. P. Loke and Y. A. L. Lim, "Helminths and the microbiota: parts of the hygiene hypothesis," *Parasite Immunology* 37, no. 6 (June 2015): 314–23, doi:10.1111/pim.12193.
10. Henry J. McSorley et al., "Suppression of Inflammatory Immune Responses in Celiac Disease by Experimental Hookworm Infection," *PLoS ONE (Social Psychiatry Collection)* 6, no. 9 (September 2011), doi:10.1371/journal.pone.0024092; J. Croese et al., "A proof of concept study establishing *Necator americanus* in Chron's patients and reservoir donors," *Gut* 55, no. 1 (January 2006): 136–7, doi:10.1136/gut.2005.079129; Birhanu Ayelign et al., "Helminth Induced Immunoregulation and Novel Therapeutic Avenue of Allergy," *Journal of Asthma and Allergy* 13 (2020): 439–51, doi:10.2147/JAA.S273556; M. A. Pineda et al., "Lessons from helminth infections: ES-62

highlights new interventional approaches in rheumatoid arthritis," *Clinical & Experimental Immunology* 177, no. 1 (July 2014): 13–23, doi:10.1111/cei.12252.

11. Jacques Delarue et al., "Fish Oil Prevents the Adrenal Activation Elicited by Mental Stress in Healthy Men," *Diabetes & Metabolism* 29, no. 3 (June 2003): 289–95, doi:10.1016/s1262-3636(07)70039-3.

12. Andrea J. Braakhuis, Rohith Nagulan, and Vaughan Somerville, "The Effect of MitoQ on Aging-Related Biomarkers: A Systematic Review and Meta-Analysis," *Oxidative Medicine and Cellular Longevity* (2018), doi:10.1155/2018/8575263; Toan Pham et al., "MitoQ and CoQ10 supplementation mildly suppresses skeletal muscle mitochondrial hydrogen peroxide levels without impacting mitochondrial function in middle-aged men," *European Journal of Applied Physiology* 120 (2020): 1657–69, doi:10.1007/s00421-020-04396-4.

13. Franchesca D. Choi et al., "Oral Collagen Supplementation: A Systematic Review of Dermatological Applications," *Journal of Drugs in Dermatology* 18, no. 1 (January 2019): 9–16; Kristine L. Clark et al., "24-Week study on the use of collagen hydrolysate as a dietary supplement in athletes with activity-related joint pain," *Current Medical Research and Opinion* 24, no. 5 (May 2008): 1485–96, doi:10.1185/030079908x291967.

14. Elsury Pérez et al., "Neighbourhood community life and health: A systematic review of reviews," *Health & Place* 61 (2020): 102238, doi:10.1016/j.healthplace.2019.102238; A. G. Christen, "Developing a social support network system to enhance mental and physical health," *Dental Clinics of North America* 30 (October 1986).

## Chapter 12

1. Marily Oppezzo and Daniel L. Schwartz, "Give Your Ideas Some Legs: The Positive Effect of Walking on Creative Thinking," *Journal of Experimental Psychology: Learning, Memory, and Cognition* 40, no. 4 (2014): 1142–52, doi:10.1037/a0036577; Atsunori Ariga and Alejandro Lleras, "Brief and rare mental 'breaks' keep you focused: deactivation and reactivation of task goals preempt vigilance decrements," *Cognition* 118, no. 3 (March 2011): 439–43, doi:10.1016/j.cognition.2010.12.007.

2. M. F. Scheier and C. S. Carver, "Dispositional optimism and physical health: A long look back, a quick look forward," *American Psychologist* 73, no. 9 (2018): 1082–94, doi:10.1037/amp0000384.

3. Anneli Jefferson, Lisa Bortolotti, and Bojana Kuzmanovic, "What is unrealistic optimism?" *Consciousness and Cognition* 50 (2017): 3–11, doi:10.1016/j.concog.2016.10.005.

4. Pedro Mateos-Aparicio and Antonio Rodríguez-Moreno, "The Impact of Studying Brain Plasticity," *Frontiers in Cellular Neuroscience* (February 27, 2019), doi:10.3389/fncel.2019.00066.

# Index

# About the Author

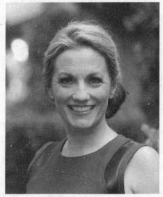

*Photo by SoulSparked*

**Dr. Donielle Wilson** is a Naturopathic Doctor, natural health expert, certified professional midwife, certified nutrition specialist, and author of *The Stress Remedy*. She graduated from Bastyr University in 2000. Dr. Doni created her Stress Recovery Protocol™ to solve her migraines and health challenges. For more than 22 years, she has helped thousands of patients overcome health challenges and achieve wellness by using specific strategies that address the whole body and ultimately resolve the underlying causes of distress. She loves teaching patients to know what they need to move from stress to thriving, live well, and do what they love with ease. Dr. Doni brings awareness to the impact of stress on our health and to the strategies and solutions for stress recovery through the media and at public and professional events. You can find articles, other resources, her podcast *How Humans Heal*, her Self C.A.R.E.™ program, and her online store at DoctorDoni.com.

## LOOKING FOR MORE SUPPORT RECOVERING FROM STRESS BASED ON YOUR STRESS TYPE?

Visit DoctorDoni.com for more
information and resources
to help you master your stress
and reset your health.

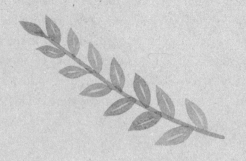